HOMEBIRTH

and other alternatives to hospital

SHEILA KITZINGER

HOMEBIRTH

and other alternatives to hospital

Photography by Marcia May

DORLING KINDERSLEY
London · New York · Stuttgart

A DORLING KINDERSLEY BOOK

Editor
LINDY NEWTON

Senior Editor
CAROLYN RYDEN

Art Editors
SALLY McKAY
SARAH SCRUTTON

Managing Editor
DAPHNE RAZAZAN

Managing Art Editor
ANNE-MARIE BULAT

First published in Great Britain in 1991
by Dorling Kindersley Limited,
9 Henrietta Street, London WC2E 8PS

A CIP catalogue record for this book is available from the
British Library

ISBN 0-86318-616-5

Typeset by SX Composing Ltd
Reproduced by Chroma Graphics (Overseas) Pte Ltd
Printed and bound by Amadeus Ltd, Italy

CONTENTS

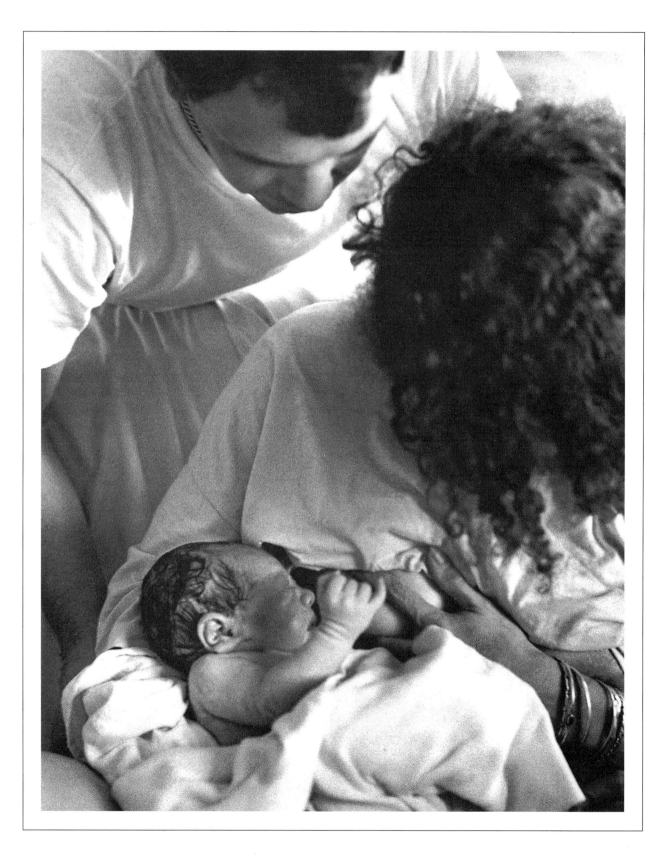

1

Why Birth Without Hospital?

Having a baby is one of the most important passages in your life. You feel the child develop and move inside you; in labour you swim with contractions that are like tidal waves sweeping through your body; as you push the baby down, you know the intensity of the birth passion, and then reach out with eager hands to welcome your baby and cradle this new life in your arms. To see love made flesh is to witness a miracle.

CHOICES ABOUT CHILDBIRTH

Whether birth is difficult or easy, painful or pain-free, long-drawn-out or brief, it need not be a medical event. It should never be conducted as if it were no more than a tooth extraction. For childbirth has much deeper significance than the removal of a baby like a decayed molar from a woman's body. The dawning of consciousness in a human being who is opening eyes for the first time on our world is packed with meaning for the mother and father, and can be also for everyone who shares in this greatest adventure of all.

At least, that is how many women see birth. Not all of us, of course. There are women who think too much fuss is made about the birth experience, and who simply want it to be painless and over with as soon as possible so that they can get on with their lives. That is a valid point of view. Some women are happy to accept induction, an epidural, and a forceps delivery, or a planned Caesarean section, and feel more secure knowing that childbirth is being managed by a top obstetrician with skills that augment or replace the natural process. I believe that women should be able to have what they choose in childbirth. It is our bodies to which this is happening, and other people should not make decisions for us or make us feel guilty because they would have chosen a different way.

"It's the difference between nurses rushing past you in the corridor, in a place where you don't belong, and inviting people into your home, the place that belongs to you."

There are many other women, however, who hope for childbirth in which they, not the doctors, are in control. They want to have the information that will enable them to make their own decisions, to prepare themselves for an experience in which they participate fully, and do not wish labour and birth to be taken over by managers.

They know that it is easier to do this on their own ground, in a place to which the doctors and midwives who are their caregivers come as guests. They would like to give birth outside hospital. This may be either in their own home, or in a birth centre in which the rhythms of a labouring woman's body are honoured and waited on, and where birth is non-interventionist and centred on people instead of on mechanical processes.

Hospitals exist where all members of staff share this attitude, but they are few and far between. You need only one person who is out of tune with such ideas, who believes in the aggressive management of labour, who, instead of being client-oriented, sees a woman as a patient who must obey hospital protocols, one person who is anxious and afraid, and who cannot trust women's bodies, for the environment in which birth takes place to be poisoned, and completely unsuitable for the focused concentration and inner confidence that is needed for a good birth.

WHAT IS A "GOOD BIRTH"?

A good birth is not just a matter of safety, or of achieving the goal of a live and physically healthy mother and baby. We want birth to be as safe as we can make it, but should not take it for granted that delivery in an operating theatre is necessarily the best way to achieve this. Childbirth has to do with emotions as well as with the sheer mechanics of descent, rotation, and delivery. It is bound to be so, because it is a major transition in the life of the mother, the father, and the whole family. Everything that happens in birth influences the way in which a woman perceives herself afterwards. It can affect the relationship between her and the baby, and between both parents and their baby, for years to come. Women have written to me to seek help with their intensely negative feelings about births that occurred 30 or 40 years earlier, and in an attempt to exorcise finally the self-hatred, guilt, and alienation that they experienced from then on.

A good birth is one which the woman looks back on, whatever happened, with satisfaction and fulfilment. Birth can be a positive experience even when, for reasons that cannot be avoided, there is a great deal of pain, or sometimes grieving. I have known a woman labour with a baby who she knew had already died. She was nurtured by her partner's loving support and, mingled with the agony of loss, there was an awareness that the experience was tender, compassionate, and profound.

Women who give birth at home, or in a place that they themselves have created in a birth centre or small hospital, believe that this offers the best environment for birth for themselves and their babies. It is far from being a selfish or thoughtless choice: working towards this kind of birth, and often struggling for it, entails much self-searching, questioning, and negotiation.

Reasons for choosing an out-of-hospital birth

Time and again, in discussions I have had with women about their reasons for choosing to give birth at home or in a birth centre rather than a hospital, the same priorities emerge:

☐ Having a relaxed, peaceful atmosphere for labour and birth.

☐ Feeling the security and comfort of a familiar environment.

☐ Knowing that she is free to be herself throughout the whole process of giving birth, to do whatever she feels like doing, to move around as she wishes, to give birth in any position she chooses, and to make any noises that come spontaneously.

In the first hour after birth a baby is alert and responsive, so is much more interesting to meet than a bundle in a cot.

☐ Having no interventions at all, either high-tech obstetric ones, or others that are often done routinely in hospitals, such as artificial rupture of the membranes.

☐ Being able to labour without drugs of any kind, and to explore other ways of handling pain.

☐ Knowing that those caring for her are her guests rather than managers, and that they make decisions together, instead of decisions being imposed on her.

☐ Enjoying a relationship of equality with those caring for her.

☐ Having a midwife birth rather than an obstetric delivery.

☐ Sharing intimately with others who are close to her; enjoying the sense of loving community.

☐ Keeping the family together; having the other children there or close by.

☐ Avoiding an episiotomy and perhaps achieving an intact perineum.

☐ Never being separated from the baby.

☐ Having the kind of nurturing after birth that is personal and intimate and very different from being in an institution.

Women who feel that they can retain control over what is happening to them during the birth, who understand the options available, and are consulted about what they prefer, are much more likely to experience birth as satisfying than those who are merely at the receiving end of care, however kindly that care. When birth is disempowering, a woman feels degraded, abused, and mutilated.* But, when birth is empowering, the experience is enriching, her self-confidence is enhanced, and she has a sense of triumph, *however difficult the labour was.*

When I studied women's experiences of epidurals,* I found that women who felt free from any pressure to have one, who were able to obtain the information they wanted and could share in decision-making, were much more likely to feel positive about the birth than those who were under pressure to have an epidural and who felt deprived of autonomy in childbirth. As one woman put it: "I was helpless, treated like a side of meat, moved, examined, and catheterized without consultation as though my labour now belonged to the doctors." In contrast, women for whom the decision to accept the offer of an epidural was one expression of their autonomy in childbirth, rather than a consequence of powerlessness and despair, have said, "I felt in control," or "I felt marvellous. I had gone from feeling and behaving like a caged wild animal to being myself, a rational human being." So a central issue in women's birth experiences is that of control: whether we can maintain control over what happens to our bodies, or whether control is taken from us.

To explore all the options about the place of birth, to decide on birth at home or in a birth centre of your choice, to plan ahead to have the kind of birth you want in an environment which you control yourself, to have people you love around you, to take responsibility, to prepare together with your caregivers for the best possible experience in an out-of-hospital setting, is, above all, empowering.

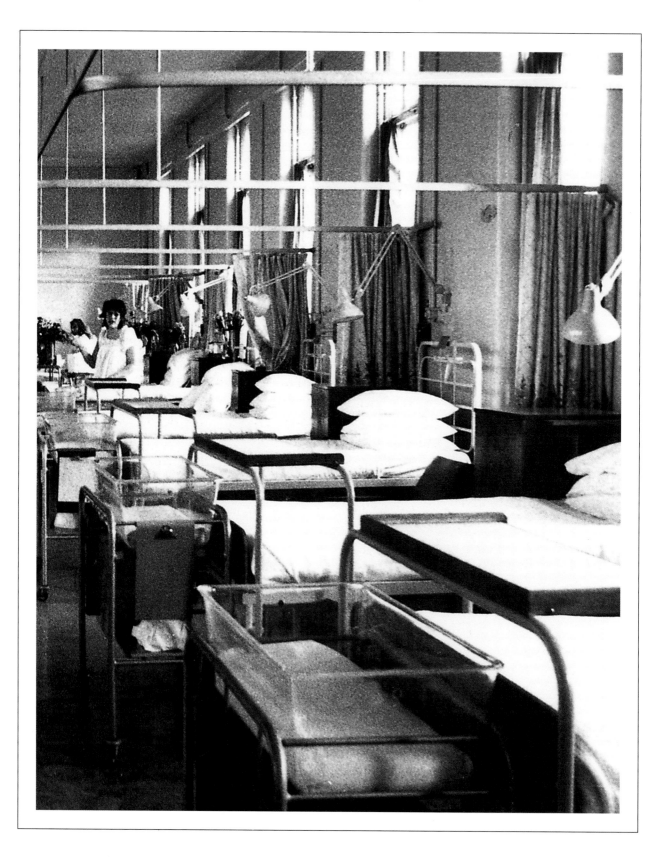

2

What's Wrong with Hospitals?

One reason why you may be considering birth outside hospital is that you have heard from other women about their unhappy experiences, have visited the hospital and did not like the atmosphere, or have already had a hospital birth and are determined not to repeat the experience. The same hospital that offers superb care to people who are ill may provide an environment for the natural physiological function of childbirth that introduces unnecessary risks, obstructs the normal physiological process, and inculcates in women who are giving birth anxiety, dependency, fear, and loss of self-confidence.

THE HOSPITAL SYSTEM

The maternity hospitals of the 18th and 19th centuries were created as charity institutions for poor women who had nowhere else to go and for unmarried women bearing their babies in shame. Other women gave birth at home. These institutions provided raw material for obstetric practice, and women were used to demonstrate obstetrics and gynaecology to medical students. They were guinea pigs for research too. The first experiments for artificially inducing labour were conducted on poor women who could not afford doctors' fees and who entered hospital as clinic patients.

In the United States poor women without health insurance still provide a pool of patients on whom students can learn. In Britain women having babies in teaching hospitals may find medical students grouped round the bed, and may never discover that the doctor who laboriously stitched an episiotomy was a house officer learning how to do it for the first time.

Following the Second World War, the British National Health Service made medical care accessible to all without need to worry about payment. Many other European countries created social security and health care systems funded by tax-payers, based on the policy that health care is a national responsibility.

With the creation of the British National Health Service there also came government health policies about childbirth and where it should take place. The decision was made that there should be sufficient beds for all women to have their babies in hospital, and birth became more and more medicalized. This was happening at a time when the standard of living was rising fast. A generation of British children had grown up who had benefited from the simple, good nutrition of the war years – wholemeal bread, orange juice, milk, few fats, little meat, and high consumption of vegetables. People were healthier than ever before. As a result women were more likely to be fit during pregnancy, did not suffer from anaemia, and did not think of pregnancy as an illness. Babies were born healthier, and the perinatal mortality rate – the death of babies at and immediately after birth – dropped progressively, so that now it is at an all time low of 8 per 1,000.

Obstetricians claim that this is due to better obstetric services, and to the policy of hospital birth for all. Yet still today women who are at the bottom of the social scale, whose partners are manual workers or who are unemployed, are twice as likely to have a baby who dies as middle class women. Social differences – education, general health, access to information, housing conditions, nutrition, attitudes to smoking, and ease of communication between caregivers and patients – have a powerful effect on the perinatal mortality rate. Babies die and women suffer in childbirth and afterwards because of poverty and neglect.

Sophisticated equipment, modern, high-technology machines, anaesthetists and doctors with surgical skills are available only in hospital, of course. This equipment and these skills can be life-saving – for a small minority of babies. But increasingly researchers are asking whether the intervention that takes place, often routinely, in many hospital births may not be hazardous. Most of these techniques have been introduced without adequate research. The question is whether procedures such as induction of labour, stimulation of the uterus with drugs once labour has started, artificial rupture of the membranes, the use of large quantities of pain-killing drugs, and continuous electronic monitoring of the fetus may not be harmful for mothers and babies if they take place as a matter of routine and are not used *selectively*.

Hospital ritual

The trouble is that almost every woman going into hospital today finds that procedures she does not wish to have are mandatory because of hospital protocols about care and rules laid down by obstetricians. These include interventions such as having the waters broken when the cervix is 3–4 cm dilated; having to conform to a pattern of 1 cm dilatation per hour in labour – otherwise having an intravenous drip inserted in the arm and a uterine stimulant dripped into the bloodstream; and regulations such as being allowed only two hours, or an hour and a half, or an hour, or even 45 minutes, to deliver following full dilatation – before being given a forceps delivery or vacuum extraction because "the baby is at risk".

There are more subtle interventions too; things that affect the atmosphere in which birth takes place and the attitudes of everyone participating. They include having to put on a hospital gown, being put to bed as if you were ill, not being able to eat and drink when you want to, the constant checking of the progress of labour against the clock, being surrounded by strangers who talk over you and about you, rather than to you, being treated like an irresponsible child who is not given any control, and the whole emphasis on pathology – detecting things that might go wrong – instead of on supporting the spontaneous flow of labour.

These interventions can lead to a massive loss of confidence in a woman. She is expected to be passive and obedient – a "good patient". She comes to distrust her body. She may feel alienated from everything that is happening to her, and this although caregivers are trying to be kind. They may be unaware of how she is feeling and of the distress that is bottled up inside

"I was very grateful that there was no question of tampering with me, no enemas, no shaving, no cutting, no drugs; we were both so thankful not to have to waste energy in arguing the toss over any of these things."

her, to emerge only later, days, weeks, or months after the baby is born. She is likely to believe that all her negative emotions about the birth, and the way in which it is replayed over and over again in her mind, and sometimes too, the hostility that bursts through towards her baby, are her own fault, and she feels terribly guilty.

NEW DEVELOPMENTS

Astonishing changes in obstetrics and in women's attitudes to childbirth occurred through the 70s and 80s. A new partnership between obstetrics and electronic engineering opened up windows on the womb with ultrasound; technological innovations made birth more complicated, compelling the mother to be a passive patient; and birth was seen by obstetricians as a medical event that could take place only in an intensive care setting equipped to meet all possible disasters. At the same time, women in almost every industrialized country have been clamouring for care that is more humane, more personal, more sensitive to their needs, seeking an environment in which they can be in tune with the spontaneous psycho-biological processes of birth and with the creative energy pouring through their bodies.

The result has been, on the one hand, more and more obstetric intervention and, on the other, a reformation movement in which women are rediscovering the value of small-scale, low-tech birthplaces, seeking alternative settings such as birthing centres and birth rooms, and even, in spite of intense opposition from the medical system, making the decision to give birth in their own homes.

During the 80s there were also exciting developments in many British and other European hospitals because of pressure from women to provide a user-friendly maternity service, and mothers and midwives got together to discuss changes that could be made and how they might work better together. The result was that midwives, and in many hospitals obstetricians too, sought to create a more humane and caring environment for birth. In country after country shaving of the perineum and the routine use of enemas or suppositories have all but disappeared. Women are encouraged to walk about throughout the first stage of labour and midwives – and more rarely obstetricians – allow mothers to be in any position which is comfortable for them to give birth. Birth plans have been introduced. Women are asked what they would like, and caregivers are listening more to their patients, and recording their wishes in the case-notes. All this is to be warmly welcomed. We are making progress.

"It isn't a matter of what it looks like. The hospital birthing rooms are all chintzy. But the staff decide what you do and when you do it. They're in control. I don't want to be 'managed' by anybody."

One question to resolve is, "Will birth in this place be both safe and empowering for me as a woman?"

Even so, hospitals are *institutions* – and often very large, complex, bureaucratic, and hierarchically organized institutions. They have to be managed so that the different parts of the whole structure can work together efficiently. Under these circumstances it is easy to abrogate responsibility and for an individual's main concern to be to oil the wheels of the system and to make it run smoothly. It is not surprising that women's needs and wishes are often ignored or trivialized. Hospitals would function much more efficiently if there were no patients.

On hospital territory patients may be allowed choice, but they have no real power. The territory belongs to the hospital management. When I analysed the words and phrases used by 40 women who had given birth at home and compared their accounts with 40 others by women who all delivered vaginally in hospital, I found that many of those in hospital used words such as "allowed" or "let me", but that no home birth mothers used these words. Although many hospital birth mothers felt very positive about their experience, they did not have the same sense of being able to control what happened to them.

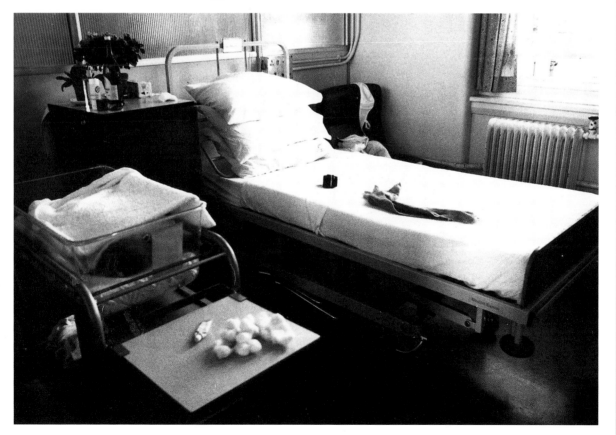

THE EFFECTS OF STRESS

Labour is stressful for most women, even in an out-of-hospital setting where they feel safe, confident, and among friends. In hospital, environmental stress is added to this psychological stress.

Hospital birth is often very stressful because a woman is in a strange place, she has to cope with a number of different professionals who care for her, and the emphasis is on things that may go wrong. It is not simply a matter of pain. This added stress combines with the stress from the pain, and a woman becomes *distressed*. Distress tends to interfere with the efficiency of uterine action, and labour slows down or the woman is unable to push her baby out. Because it interferes with the physiology of birth, this excessive stress may affect the condition of the baby before and after birth.

When under stress our bodies produce catecholamines, or "stress hormones", the best-known of which are adrenalin and noradrenalin. This is normal and advantageous under most circumstances, because cathecholamines help the body adjust to stress. If the stress is excessive, however, or goes on for too long, the body exhausts its resources and can no longer adjust to the stress.

When catecholamine levels rise abnormally in a woman in labour, her uterus contracts less efficiently, contractions become weaker or spasmodic, dilatation of the cervix is slower, and labour longer.* Sometimes the uterus simply stops contracting for a while. This often occurs when a woman first arrives in hospital, even when contractions have been strong and regular at home. The rise in catecholamine levels has the effect of making her more anxious, which also means that she feels more pain. This in turn further increases catecholamine levels. It is a vicious circle.

However, when there is no added stress, the hard work of labour, the mother's excitement, the mobilization of her energy to meet the challenge of contractions as they get stronger, longer, and closer together, are good for the baby. The fetus also makes its own catecholamines and, when these are at a normal level, they push up production of prostaglandins and stimulate oxygen uptake. Blood is shunted from near the skin surface to the baby's vital organs – the heart, brain, and liver – and energy stores are mobilized ready for birth. Catecholamines protect the fetus from the effects of a reduced flow of blood through the placenta at the height of contractions. They also help the baby adjust to life outside the uterus by facilitating absorption of liquid in the lungs, by enabling the baby to generate its own heat, and by producing the alert, attentive state that helps parents fall in love with their baby.

"I have just had my first baby at home. It was an incredible experience – the equivalent of climbing Mount Everest."
A doctor

But catecholamines are pushed above this physiological level when the mother is under great stress during labour, with the result that less oxygenated blood flows to her uterus and through the placenta to her baby. The baby compensates by increasing its own production of catecholamines to excessive levels, with resulting fetal heart irregularities due to lack of oxygen.

Very high catecholamine levels may lead to problems for the newborn baby too: breathing difficulties; difficulty in regulating his temperature so that he becomes very cold; reduction in plasma volume (the liquid part of blood); metabolic acidosis (disturbance in the chemical balance of blood); jaundice (excess bile pigment in blood); and even necrotizing enterocolitis (diarrhoea with blood in the faeces).

Obstetric anaesthetists who are concerned about the effect of high catecholamine levels on babies respond by recommending that small hospitals and GP units should be closed, all women moved to large regional hospitals, and as many offered epidural anaesthesia as the epidural service can handle.* An epidural can provide blessed relief when a woman is in uncontrollable pain. But often the pain is actually being caused, or made uncontrollable, by the way she is being treated. The hospital environment, with its rules, tests, and constant threat of obstetric intervention, is pushing up both her catecholamine levels and those of her baby.

HOW HOSPITAL BIRTH CAN BE DANGEROUS

"When a woman is at home and you want to intervene, it forces you to think whether it's really necessary. The very ease with which interventions take place in hospital increases the risk of them being performed unnecessarily."
An obstetrician

Hospitals are often dangerous places in which to give birth. It is usually taken for granted that they must be safe because they have the equipment and skilled staff to deal with medical emergencies. But sometimes they are the cause of these emergencies in the first place. Many interventions that take place routinely in hospital birth are iatrogenic. That is, they result in illness produced by doctors.

Induction

The artificial start of labour, induction is done in one, or a combination, of three ways:

☐ Synthetic oxytocin is introduced into the woman's bloodstream.

☐ Prostaglandin in the form of a gel is placed in the cervix.

☐ Amniotomy is performed – the water bubble in which the baby lies is broken with an instrument resembling a crochet hook or small forceps.

The practice of induction and the exact method of doing it vary widely in different countries and between different obstetricians. In the United States the FDA has not licensed prostaglandin for induction of labour, for instance, so synthetic oxytocin – pitocin – is used. Rates of induction vary radically too. When a comparative study was done on European countries in the 70s, the induction rate in Norway was found to be about 10 per cent, whereas in England and Wales it was 40 per cent.* In the UK women often did not even know why their labours were being induced, and they were rarely asked for their informed consent. It was the doctor's decision, and the mother was expected to go along with it for the sake of her baby.

Women protested at this high rate of induction, and obstetricians discovered that it had disastrous consequences for both mothers and babies. Babies were being pushed out into the world before they were ready for life, and special care nurseries were filled with babies who were premature because they had been induced.* At present the induction rate in the UK is about one in four. This is still much too high, on the grounds of both safety and the mother's comfort.

Pros and cons of induction

A doctor may want to induce if a woman goes two weeks, ten days, or even a few days, past her due date. Some like to induce at term – on or around the expected date – on the grounds that "this is a very precious baby", especially with an older mother. Many obstetricians find it difficult to live with the uncertainty of when labour will start, and there are women who prefer to know exactly when the birth will be. This accounts for many of the social inductions that take place, though these inductions for convenience are often disguised as being medically indicated.

In the UK the induction epidemic of the 70s resulted in fewer and fewer births taking place at weekends and on public holidays.* When obstetricians were interviewed about induction, half of them said that it had improved their job satisfaction and made the running of maternity departments easier.*

Induction, like all other interventions, can be useful in selected situations: if a woman has pre-eclampsia, for example, and her blood pressure is dangerously high, the placenta may fail to support the baby's life, and it may be safer to deliver the baby early. A diabetic woman's baby tends to grow very large and, though premature, may be more safely delivered early.

But induction is not always successful and always has risks. Much of the research that has been done has ignored these risks.

□ An induced labour is often fast and furious, so is more painful than one that starts naturally. In my own study of some women's experiences of induced labour* I found that when women whose second labour was induced compared this with the previous labour which had not been induced, two-thirds of them said that the second labour was more painful, though as a rule second labours are less painful.

"The pain was shocking – double-peaked contractions that lasted almost two minutes. I hadn't wanted an epidural, but there was no way I could have managed without one."

□ Because induction is often given in a package deal with epidural anaesthesia, other interventions may take place which add new risks with a knock-on effect. Having a catheter inserted in the bladder increases the risk of infection, for example. Being immobilized makes it more likely that dilatation is slow, and so the drip is turned up and more artificial oxytocin is fed into the bloodstream. Large quantities of fluid may produce water intoxication. A woman who drinks as much fluid as she wants during labour does not take too much. But, if fluids are introduced through an intravenous drip, her metabolism is altered and, if she receives an excessive quantity, she may suffer convulsions, and even coma. When oxytocin is being dripped into a woman's bloodstream in addition to glucose solution, she is further at risk of water intoxication.

□ The uterus may become hypertonic. That is, it may clamp down on the baby with very strong contractions lasting two minutes or longer, and this reduces the flow of blood. In normal labour contractions squeeze the baby as if it were being hugged tightly. Blood flow is lessened at the height of contractions but increased as each one finishes. In induced labour there is a risk that this rhythm is lost and that the uterus goes into spasm. The result is that the baby's heartbeat becomes either very fast – tachycardia – or slow – bradycardia. At birth the baby may need resuscitation and be taken to the special care nursery for observation.

"They ruptured my membranes, set up a glucose drip, and put a scalp electrode on the baby's head, I felt trapped. Then they added syntocinon to the drip and gave me pethidine."

□ It is impossible to move about freely, or sometimes even to change position in bed with ease. The woman has little bits of plastic, wire, and rubber sticking out all over her: an intravenous drip in her arm; a blood pressure cuff encircling her upper arm; a catheter in her bladder; an electrode screwed or clipped into the baby's scalp to record its heartbeat; and a plastic tube stuck in her back and snaking up to her shoulder, where it is fixed with sticky tape so that the epidural can be topped up without having to lift her.

□ Because labour is always monitored electronically when induction takes place, warning signs in the baby's heart-rate are watched for. A worrying print-out may unfurl from the monitor, there may be flashing red lights,

"I had an intravenous drip and was strapped up to two fetal monitors. I longed to get upright, but it was impossible."

and alarm bells may be triggered. All this is distressing for a woman in labour. Then delivery may be hastened with an episiotomy – a cut to enlarge the vagina – and perhaps forceps or, if the head is still too high, a Caesarean section.

At home or in an out-of-hospital birth centre labour is not induced, for it is recognized that induction brings risks and may entail other forms of intervention, including drugs for pain relief and an assisted delivery, which are incompatible with care outside hospital. Having a baby at home is one way of ruling out entirely a whole category of risks that starts with induction, escalates with pain-killing drugs, and peaks when uterine stimulants are stepped up because the drugs have made contractions weaker or erratic.

Active management

"I was given oxytocin with no explanation. They told my husband, 'She's being a bit slow.' It was a very shocking experience."

In many hospitals today labours are managed "actively". That is, the obstetrician takes charge, with the aim of making labour conform to a norm. A typical pattern is that it should not last longer than 12 hours, dilatation should take place by at least 1 cm an hour, and delivery must occur within one hour of full dilatation.

If a labour is not conforming to this model, intravenous oxytocin is used to stimulate the uterus to greater activity, or delivery is completed with forceps, vacuum extraction, or Caesarean section.* Active management was first introduced in Dublin, where the emphasis is on a short, snappy labour, and also on one-to-one nurse care. (For some reason the Irish obstetricians who started this system ignore midwives and talk about "nurses" instead.) They call it "military efficiency with a human face".* No fathers are present. Epidurals are rarely given. Pethidine is available only in small doses. "The time of delivery is stated to within 30 minutes: a woman is told at noon that her baby is expected at four o'clock in the afternoon, give or take half an hour."* Women must labour silently: "A woman owes it to herself, to her husband, and to her child, and to every other woman *who may be unfortunate enough to labour at the same time* [my italics], to be well-briefed in this matter. The disruptive effect of one disorganized and frightened woman in a delivery unit extends far beyond her own comfort and safety, and there should be no hesitation in telling her so."

"Everything was just 'done' to me. I wasn't consulted about anything and it was all out of my control."

Mothers have a duty also to those who care for them during labour: "It should be clearly understood that nurses must not be expected to submit to the sometimes outrageous conduct of perfectly healthy women who cannot be persuaded to . . . behave with dignity and purpose during the most important hours of their lives – nor should nurses be held responsible in any way for the degrading scenes which occasionally result."* So, when a woman pleads for pain-killers, weeps in terror, or screams out in agony, these obstetricians consider that it is *her* fault.

The use of oxytocin to augment labour is not without risk. Just as when it is used for induction, labour is more painful for the mother, there may be hyperstimulation of the uterus, and the baby may become short of oxygen.

"They put me on an oxytocin drip against my will. I was left with a student who read the paper and totally ignored me."

This is why obstetricians in Dublin do not advise the use of oxytocin in multigravidae (women who have already had babies). Elsewhere, however, active management may include the routine speeding up of labour, even when the problem is not, in fact, uterine "inefficiency" but disproportion – that is, when the baby cannot pass through the mother's pelvis. Then the uterus may rupture (the muscle tears), and the baby may be squeezed so hard and often that there is shortage of oxygen – hypoxia; in some cases the baby may turn out to have cerebral palsy as a result, and the mother's pelvis may even be fractured.*

When you give birth in territory which you control, instead of management protocols dictating how labour should be conducted, you are yourself the active birth-giver. This is the fundamental difference between birth in hospital and birth at home or in the kind of birth centre where the power is yours, not the doctor's.

Electronic fetal monitoring

Many obstetricians believe that continuous electronic fetal monitoring should be employed in all labours "just in case". In hospital, monitoring is done either from the time a woman is admitted until she delivers, or a "strip" print-out is taken for about an hour after she is admitted and, if all is well, taken again only if further information is required later in the labour.

Already by 1980 almost 50 per cent of hospital births in the USA were monitored with continuous electronic fetal monitoring.* Yet there is marked disagreement between obstetricians about what ought to be done when the print-out from the monitor is different from what would normally be expected. When four experienced obstetricians studied the same fetal heart traces and were asked whether they would deliver immediately, they agreed in only one out of five cases.* Nearly two years later these obstetricians were shown the same traces again and asked what they would do. In one out of five cases they assessed them differently from the time before.

There is no evidence that electronic fetal monitoring saves babies' lives or that the condition of babies at birth has anything to do with whether or not they had electronic monitoring during labour.* It has been discovered, however, that when babies are monitored they are less likely to have neonatal seizures.* This might be a very important finding except that further studies have revealed that these seizures are not linked with any long-term problems.*

Risks of electronic monitoring

At first glance it might look as if this particular piece of high technology could do nothing but good. But the trouble is that electronic fetal monitoring itself causes problems and introduces its own risks.

☐ If monitoring is to be employed safely, caregivers must know how to use it and understand how to interpret the information correctly. This is not always the case. Sometimes the monitor picks up the mother's heartbeat rather than the baby's, for example. Since the baby's heart is normally about twice as fast as hers, it then appears as if there is fetal bradycardia. Unnecessary intervention takes place, and the baby may be delivered by forceps or Caesarean section.*

Sometimes the opposite happens: caregivers are lulled into false security when a woman is wired up to a monitor and no one bothers to check the print-out regularly or looks at the whole pattern of her labour.

The monitor cannot give birth. Only the woman can do that. The monitor records data, and what is done or not done then depends on the skills of the caregivers.

☐ Although some monitors work with radio waves – telemetry – and allow a woman to walk about, the use of most monitors means that she must stay in one place, either strapped up tightly with belts around her abdomen or wired up with a pin stuck in the baby's head. This immobilization causes unnecessary pain and may slow down contractions and make them weaker, so that dilatation is slower. Sometimes labour becomes so slow that the decision is made to augment it with an oxytocin intravenous drip.

A woman is often told to lie still so that the print-out is clear.* If she is lying on her back, not only does she get backache, but there is a danger of compression of her aorta – the large blood vessel in the lower part of her body – by her heavy uterus, with a resulting slow down in the flow of blood back to her heart. She becomes sick, dizzy, faint, and may even black out. This deprives the baby of oxygen too. The monitor then spills out ominous traces in the fetal heart-rate, recording information about a situation which it was responsible for creating in the first place.

☐ When there are staff shortages, or when staff do not understand the importance of being centred on the woman and creating a calm, loving atmosphere, a partner is often told to keep an eye on the monitor, or a nurse or midwife pops in at intervals, studies the print-out, says a cheery word to the mother, and disappears again. Attention turns to the electronic equipment rather than being focused on the woman's needs, and she loses emotional support. Even with her partner close beside her, a woman may then be isolated. An electronic monitor cannot take the place of human caring and understanding.

Mind and body are not two separate, distinct systems in childbirth. A woman's body works best when she feels confident, secure, emotionally supported, and on her own ground.

☐ An electrode can be fixed on the baby's head only after the membranes have ruptured. If this has not occurred spontaneously in early labour, an amniotomy is performed, usually at 3 or 4 cm dilatation. When there is no interference, membranes usually do not rupture at the beginning of labour, but at the very end of the first stage. Artificial rupture of the membranes interferes with the sterile environment in which the baby is contained and may result in infection. It also removes the protection provided by the water bubble which normally cushions the baby and its cord and placenta against excessive pressure, so that blood flow is impeded. The monitor may then demonstrate that the baby is in trouble, but it was the amniotomy performed in order to put the electrode on the baby's head that was responsible for the stress to the baby.

☐ Some doctors are experimenting with ways of fixing electrodes using strong suction or glue so that they do not have to harpoon the baby, but they have not yet succeeded in producing a viable alternative to scalp clips or screws. When a baby's scalp is penetrated by the hook or spiral screw, there is danger of damaging the scalp when removing it.* Sometimes there is a bald patch and hair never grows there, or a scalp abscess forms, which has to be treated with antibiotics.*

☐ In most hospitals the introduction of electronic fetal monitoring immediately pushes the Caesarean section rate up at least three-fold. After the equipment has been in use for some time, staff relax a bit and the rate drops again. But in industrialized countries worldwide there is a steady increase in Caesarean sections, which can be attributed partly to electronic monitoring. Caesarean section is riskier for women than vaginal birth. Five times as many women die after a Caesarean section than after a vaginal birth (50 compared with 10 per 100,000 deliveries), and there is a much increased risk of infection and other postpartum problems.*

☐ Information that the fetal monitor provides bears little or no relation to the baby's condition at birth. Too little is known about normal variations in the fetal heart-rate to warrant intervention only on the basis of a suspicious trace on an electronic monitor.

☐ Many monitors don't work well all the time. Women say that they were told: "Oh, don't take any notice of that. It isn't working properly," or a husband is advised to kick the machine when a light starts flashing because "it's always doing that. It doesn't mean anything." Yet the rule is that the woman must be attached to a monitor, even though it is not providing accurate information. This can be a very bewildering and frightening experience. Under these circumstances the monitor is worse than useless. It is dangerous.

Intermittent monitoring

The older way of monitoring the condition of the baby during labour was to listen to its heart intermittently through a trumpet-shaped fetal stethoscope. The accuracy of this method depends on how often and when it is done.

It is important to know whether the fetal heart is picking up regularly *after* contractions. The baby who is over-stressed is usually the one whose heart speeds up a lot – above 160 beats a minute – or slows down below 120 beats a minute with contractions, and *stays* high or low in the space between contractions. When the heart slows down at the peak of contractions, a perfectly natural occurrence, it is called a type 1 dip. When the heart stays slow afterwards, it is a type 2 dip. It is the type 2 dips that are worrying. If a baby is in real trouble, there are few or no variations in heart-rate. On an electronic monitor you get a flat trace.

So if a fetal stethoscope is the method of choice, it should be used at the end of every cluster of strong contractions in the late first stage, and more often in the second stage, the times in labour when contractions may be most stressful for the baby. Having a fetal stethoscope poked at you just as a contraction ends can be uncomfortable and irritating. Many women and midwives prefer a newer intermittent method of monitoring which uses Doppler ultrasound in the form of a hand-held sonic aid. This is a camera-sized instrument with a disc like a small microphone which is held over the baby's heart, registers the beats, and translates these into an audible signal – like galloping horses.

This method provides no permanent record of the heart-rate in the form of a printed trace, and this could be a disadvantage from the point of view of obstetricians anxious about possible litigation after the birth. However, litigation is very unlikely to follow a birth that has taken place, by the woman's choice, out of hospital where obstetric intervention is rare.

So high-tech gadgets may be useful, but only those that do not intrude on your ability to tune in to your own body and to the power that wells up inside you, on the full tide of which your baby is brought to birth.

The rushed second stage

Clock-watched labours are the rule in hospitals. When women describe their labours in hospital, they often refer to the time and say such things as: "My induction was well-timed to fit into working hours," "The pupil midwife told me to watch the clock and time contractions," or "The baby was posterior, and sister said they'd give me a few hours to see what happened." When women give birth at home, they talk about meal-times, sunrise, sunlight pouring through the window, sunset and night-time, but they do not usually relate everything that occurred in labour to the clock.

In my own study of the language women used in describing 40 home and 40 hospital births, three-quarters of home birth mothers said that they enjoyed not being hurried and knowing that they had plenty of time.* Only four hospital birth mothers made similar statements.

In hospital the clock is master, marking the distinction between the normal and the abnormal, the labour that can be allowed to proceed without obstetric intervention and the labour that calls for immediate intervention.

"I did a home birth and had for the first time a feeling of confidence because it was just happening. Any medical intervention would have been entirely inappropriate."
A doctor

Doctors and midwives who attend home births usually know how to watch and wait. They realize that the uterus works most effectively if a woman is in an upright or semi-upright position and can alter her position when she wants. They know that moving around can often change malposition or malpresentation. They are aware that anxiety and fear can make it harder for a woman to open her body and push her baby out. If she is not wasting energy trying to push, and pushes only when she wants to and for only as long as she wants to, she can work with her body, instead of fighting against it.

A second stage in which you are harried and hurried is bound to be an anxious and panic-inducing ordeal. In hospital women are often coaxed or commanded to push, and instructed to hold each breath and push as hard as they possibly can, because of the time limit on the second stage.

"The doctor gave me 20 minutes to push while she got the forceps ready. It was harrowing."

In English hospitals women having their first babies (primiparae) usually are allowed only one hour from full dilatation to delivery. Some obstetricians consider that this is far too long, and limit first-time mothers to 45 minutes or even half an hour, and multiparae to 20 minutes.*

There is no evidence that reducing the length of the second stage makes labour any safer, prevents baby deaths, or produces healthier babies.* If a baby is too large to come through the mother's pelvis, there are many clinical signs, including the head staying high, lack of progress, fetal heart arrhythmia, or type 2 dips that indicate this – not the length of the second stage alone.

The mother is often encouraged to hold her breath over prolonged periods when pushing, and this can be dangerous, because it may reduce the baby's oxygen.* One problem in many hospitals is that the second stage is reckoned to start with full dilatation of the cervix. Frequent vaginal examinations result in full dilatation being assessed and noted on the case record or partogram (labour chart) immediately it is reached, or even sometimes before this. The second stage is then timed from that point. But the woman may not yet want to push. This is natural. If the baby's head is not pressing against your pelvic floor muscles, you have no spontaneous desire to push, since this is a reflex stimulated when there is pressure against nerve endings in the pelvic floor.

From that moment it is a race to the finishing post. The woman may be bullied in an effort to get the baby born before the obstetrician must be called, and with his appearance delivery is usually completed with episiotomy and forceps or vacuum extraction, or a Caesarean section.

Episiotomy

You are much more likely to have an episiotomy – a cut in the vagina to enlarge the birth opening – if you have your baby in hospital than you are if you give birth at home or in a birth centre.

Episiotomy rates vary widely between countries, and even between hospitals and different obstetricians in the same hospital. In some hospitals nine out of ten women receive an episiotomy.* Some obstetricians believe that all first-time mothers should have an episiotomy. They may believe, too, that any woman who has had an episiotomy should have one with the next delivery, because scar tissue must be present that will not stretch to let the baby out easily. The result is that everyone has an episiotomy except those who deliver too fast to have one.

Pros and cons of episiotomy

Episiotomy is performed with the aim of saving the baby from being "battered" against the mother's pelvic floor, to prevent damage to these muscles, to avoid injury to her anus, to prevent later stress incontinence (leaking of urine), and to achieve better healing than after laceration with "a nice clean cut that is easier to sew up than a nasty, jagged tear". There is no evidence that episiotomy does any of these things.* Even if it did not matter what happened to the mother and if episiotomies were performed for the baby's sake alone, the claim that episiotomy protects the baby's head or produces a baby in better condition is not supported by the evidence.*

Because obstetricians make rules as to how long their patients may be in the second stage, midwives and junior doctors delivering babies with no obstetrician present perform episiotomies to hasten delivery if they come up against that time limit.*

Although occasionally the baby's head can be nicked by scissors, the hazards of episiotomy generally concern the mother, not the baby, in a number of ways:

☐ Having an episiotomy is often acutely painful. If it is performed at the height of a contraction when the perineum is stretched and bulging, a woman may not feel it. But, because of possible damage to the baby's head, in hospitals there are rules about it being done only between contractions. A local anaesthetic is often – not always – given first, but this itself hurts in a very sensitive place, and in many hospitals staff do not wait the three or four minutes necessary for the perineum to be fully numb before cutting.*

☐ Repair of an episiotomy is often painful. The wound must be sutured carefully, correctly aligning damaged tissues. Inadequate local anaesthesia may be used, or an area is not numbed at all, or the person doing the suturing may not wait for the anaesthetic to take effect. So perineal repair is for some women more painful than anything they experienced during the birth – much more painful than contractions or the delivery.

☐ The area is often bruised. This may be because the baby's head has been bumping against it, but the most severe bruising results from an episiotomy made too early, before the head is on the perineum. This is regular practice in some hospitals, on the grounds that in this way any stress caused by the baby's head is prevented. The scissors used may be blunt, so that they crush as well as cut the tissues, and extensive bruising results then, too.

☐ Blood loss with episiotomy may cause anaemia and make a woman feel very weak and tired, and this at a time when she wants to be alert to get to know her baby. The combination of exhaustion and pain is very demoralizing and makes a frightening start to motherhood.

☐ Many episiotomy wounds become infected, and sometimes a perineal abscess results. This is terribly painful. Infection is more common in hospital than at home, and many hospital bacteria are now penicillin resistant. Infection delays healing and, when the wound does at last heal, there may be scar tissue.

☐ Although episiotomies are performed in the theory that to make a deliberate cut prevents a tear into the anus and rectum, a third-degree laceration (fourth-degree in the USA), this occurs more often when an episiotomy has been performed than when a tear occurs naturally. A small proportion of women have an episiotomy plus a laceration, because the cut has then gone on to tear. The intricate embroidery that has to be done when this happens may entail general anaesthesia and can take a long time. The woman is in far more pain afterwards than after a second-degree laceration.*

☐ In the week after a woman's perineum has been sutured, as healing takes place, she is likely to be in constant discomfort, and in acute pain when she empties her bladder or bowels, walks, shifts position in bed, or lifts and feeds her baby. Women on postnatal wards shuffle around, bent forward, knees together, trying to cope with this pain. The second, third, and fourth days are often the worst, and then things become easier. The pain after a first-degree tear – a nick in the skin only – is much less than that after an episiotomy, which corresponds to a second-degree tear, cutting into muscle.*

Pain often lasts for some months, with a knot of scar tissue at the lower end of the vagina which may be too painful to touch. At three months postpartum a large percentage of women still have pain some of the time: if they sit down on a hard chair without thinking, wear trousers that are tight on the crotch, stand too long, or move carelessly. Women whose periods have returned say that they cannot possibly use tampons.*

The reason for this is that suturing has been done too tightly, not allowing for the swelling that follows injury to tissue that is especially sensitive. If you have ever seen anyone with a wasp sting near the eye, you know how enormous the swelling is. Perineal tissue is similar.

After an episiotomy it is impossible to have intercourse until everything has healed.* At three months more women who have had episiotomies have pain with attempted intercourse than do those who have had even severe tears. Those still in most pain are women who have had both an episiotomy and a tear.* A woman who cannot bear the thought of love-making because she is in pain often feels that it must be her fault.

A small proportion of women, even after painstaking suturing, are left with a recto-vaginal fistula (a gap in the wall between the rectum and vagina) and pass faeces through the vagina. So they have another operation weeks or months later for this to be repaired. The emotional as well as the

"My husband is very patient and understanding but he thinks I should be better by now."

30

physical effect of all this cannot be underestimated. They feel mutilated, abused, and dirty. They may feel scalding anger or be deeply depressed.

Some women have pain that continues for years. Sometimes this happens because the vagina is too tight, with the tissues stretched and aching. Sometimes nerves have been sliced through. Sometimes a large knob of scar tissue remains painful, and the woman feels as if she is sitting on thorns. When she seeks help, she may be advised to lubricate the painful area, be told that the pain will pass eventually, be sent to a psychotherapist or marriage counsellor, or be offered surgery to cut out scar tissue and improve the "cosmetic" result.

In home births and birth centres episiotomies are not done automatically. They are reserved for those situations in which a baby needs to be born quickly. Midwives have skills of "guarding" the perineum with a hand, enabling a woman to give birth slowly and gently, so that the perineum is not over-stressed and there is less likelihood of a tear. They use hot compresses, warm water, or oil massage to soften tissues and help them to fan out, and often words that suggest vivid opening images.* Midwives and doctors who attend home births and work in birth centres acquire or have retained these skills, and many also use new methods such as birth in water, which seems to help maintain the elasticity of a woman's perineum.

NEWBORN BABIES AS PATIENTS

In hospital the moment that babies are born, and even before birth, they are treated as patients, and subjected to a range of painful practices which cause distress and interfere with their smooth adjustment to life.

In many hospitals the first assault on babies as they are born is to suction them, by passing a tube into the nose and mouth to extract any mucus that might be in the airways. This suctioning of the baby's nasal passages and throat is especially distressing for the baby when done roughly, using a catheter rather than a suction bulb.* It may result in cardiac arrhythmia and, if the catheter touches the larynx, is likely to cause laryngeal spasm. Occasionally the herpes virus or bacteria are transferred through the suction catheter to the baby from the midwife or doctor.* Even with babies who have already passed meconium (the first contents of the bowel) – a sign that they are under stress – it is uncertain whether intubation does more good than harm.*

In some hospitals another routine is to pass a tube down into the baby's stomach to clear any gastric secretions that may be there. This scouring of the baby's gastric tract is another assault. It leads to slowing of the heart-rate and spasm of the larynx, which can interfere with the baby's whole pattern of sucking and swallowing – so that feeding is made more difficult.*

Many countries have a law that all newborn babies must receive prophylaxis against gonorrhoeal blindness, so drops are put in the eyes after delivery. These are usually silver nitrate which is intensely irritating and causes babies to close their eyes, interfering with communication between the mother and her baby in the hour following birth, the time when the baby is most likely to be in a quiet, alert state.* In fact erythromycin works better than silver nitrate* and is also effective against chlamydia (thrush), which a baby can pick up from the mother's vagina.* Silver nitrate is not effective against chlamydia.

In hospital you may have little or no control over what is put in your baby's eyes because there are often hospital protocols which do not permit choice. At home this is something you decide together with your midwife.

TENDER, LOVING CARE?

In some hospitals large numbers of babies are moved to the special care nursery, if only for observation. In many countries babies are routinely separated from their mothers anyway, isolated in a small room with a large window where a nurse glances at them occasionally, as I have seen happening in Italy, or in a large nursery under bright, fluorescent lights with dozens of other babies, as in the USA, or even in a good-sized cupboard which nurses use as a refuge where they can chat and smoke – something that I have seen in the USSR.

"Every part of me seemed to fill with what I can only describe as 'a loving ecstasy'. This intense communication was never possible in hospital immediately after birth, as the babies were not beside me. But I wonder if there it could have taken place. It was something so special I think it needed exactly the right receptive conditions on both our parts for it to happen."

Apart from the emotional deprivation caused to the mother by taking her baby away from her – the reward of all her work and striving – and the loneliness and confusion the baby may feel, this is bad practice. It can be dangerous. When babies are herded together in this way, the risk of cross-infection is high, and no one is likely to watch a newborn baby as unceasingly and with such acute observation as the mother.

Thirty years after research on bonding between mothers and babies was first published* babies are still being treated as if they were the property of the hospital rather than the mother, and as if trained professionals were the only people who could safely assess a baby's condition and give appropriate care. When the World Health Organization enquired in 24 European countries what the usual practices were, it was revealed that in 17 countries babies were automatically separated from their mothers for a period of time after birth.*

"I knew they were watching me to see if we were bonding. But the birth had been such an ordeal I needed time. I couldn't be rushed. I felt I had to put on an act."

"I want to spend time with the baby and my husband, talking about the whole experience and our feelings, without a time limit and without interference – in my own familiar surroundings."

Bonding is often seen as something that must be aggressively "facilitated" or actively taught by staff, rather than as a process that cannot be rushed, that occurs in its own way and its own sweet time if a mother has her baby with her whenever she wants, for as long as she wants, and if she herself is in a supportive, friendly environment.

In some hospitals bonding theory has been incorporated into care in very destructive ways. Women say they feel they have to put on a performance and respond to their babies in the correct, loving style, because they are aware that they are under the scrutiny of staff checking to see if bonding is taking place.

Being forced to take what amounts to an examination in motherhood within a few hours or even minutes of your baby's birth is not the best way of starting off a relationship. It interferes with the powerful emotions that may be sweeping through you, and is likely to make you self-conscious, self-questioning and inhibited. Most women overcome these obstacles. But it is hard on those who have had a stressful and difficult birth, and who may not be able to "come back into themselves" and feel secure enough to reach out to their babies. They need peace and quiet, and to be nurtured themselves, before they can nurture their babies.

Many hospitals in the West have incorporated "gentle birth" or "Leboyer birth" into their practice. Lights are dimmed for delivery, voices hushed, the baby is handled gently, and given to the mother immediately. She can cuddle her newborn against her bare skin under a special heater or a blanket which covers them both, and mother, father, and baby have uninterrupted time together for about an hour after delivery.

So far, so good. But what mothers often don't realize is that the baby may then be taken from them to another place for a paediatric examination. This is a brightly lit, noisy nursery – a very different environment from the close intimacy of that first postnatal hour.

Only at home, or in a birth centre in which there is no separation between mother and baby, can a woman be sure that her healthy baby remains with her, within sight even if not in her arms, and will never be taken away from her for any reason whatever, unless she wishes it. She watches her baby intently, fascinated by each tiny movement, listens to the strange and sometimes quick, dancing patterns of breathing. What is happening is important in the development of the relationship between mother and baby in ways that we do not yet fully understand. To interfere with or destroy that intimacy is to risk interrupting a vital psychological process that may reduce the woman's confidence in herself as a mother and interfere with the flow of communication between her and her baby.

BIRTH CONTRASTS

Obstetric way of birth	Women's way of birth
Cultural definition of birth	
Potentially pathological process	Social event
Illness	Normal part of women's lives
Birth is work of doctors/nurses/midwives and other experts	Birth is work by the woman and her family and kin
The woman is a patient	The woman is a person passing through a major life transition
The setting for birth	
Hospital, territory alien to the woman	Home or other familiar surroundings
Bureaucratic, hierarchical system of care	Informal system of care
May be distant from woman's home	In a woman's home or near
Woman is separated from those close to her	With other women of neighbourhood and family
Discontinuity of care, e.g. shift changes/ woman is moved from one room or one ward to another	Continuity of care
Woman may not be free to change position and move about	Woman free to change position and move about
Caregivers: the support they give and the conduct of labour	
Young and older women who have often not themselves had babies, under direction of male obstetricians	Older and more experienced women who are themselves mothers
Trained to focus on medical aspects of birth	See birth as holistic process
Professional care that is authoritarian	Shared decision-making between caregivers and woman giving birth

Obstetric way of birth	Women's way of birth
Caregivers (continued)	
Often class distinction between obstetricians and patients	No class distinction between caregivers and woman giving birth
Dominant-subordinate relationship	Equal relationship
Information about health, disease, and degree of risk kept secret	Information shared
Care depersonalized	Personal caring
Little emotional support	Often strong emotional support
Lack of communication	Verbal and non-verbal encouragement
Use of medical language	Familiar language and imagery used
Threatening and often punitive behaviour, e.g. commanding, scolding, warning	Empathy
Little cultural awareness of rituals, beliefs, social behaviour, values	Cultural awareness because they are part of the same culture
Spiritual aspects of birth ignored or treated as embarrassing	Awareness of spiritual significance of birth
Techniques used	
No skills to preserve the physiological progress of labour	Skills to preserve the physiological progress of labour
Obstetric intervention	Usually intervention-free
Drugs for pain relief	Comfort skills, e.g. massage, hot and cold compresses, holding
Skills and resources to handle complicated and obstructed labour, e.g. intravenous fluids, oxytocin stimulation, surgery	Few resources to handle complicated obstructed labour

This chart is based on one devised by Sandra Anderson and Frants Stangard.* I have freely adapted their model of traditional midwifery to illustrate the main differences between hospital and home birth.

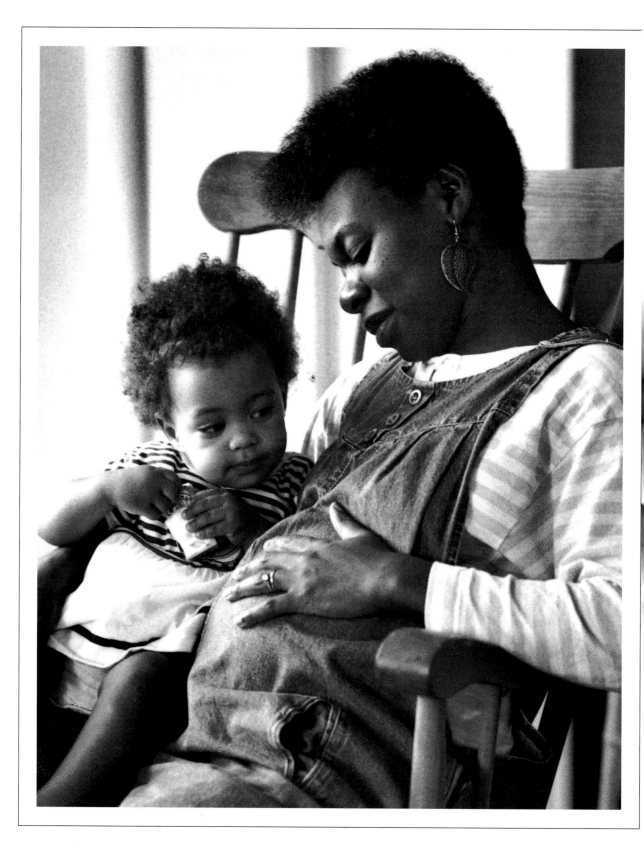

3

Making the Right Decision

Decisions about where to give birth should spring from realistic risk assessment and from your own inner values. Any woman who decides that birth without hospital is right for her in a society that is hostile to freedom in childbirth takes responsibility for weighing up the risks, and also expresses the courage of human beings to resist autocracy, dogma and the power of the medical system. Her decision is based on deeply held *values*. Doctors, however, tend to see birth exclusively in terms of *risk*.

ASSESSING RISK

"You are high risk because you are 31 . . . it is your first baby and you have an untried pelvis . . . you had a miscarriage last year . . . you are in a high-risk ethnic group . . . you are single . . . this is your fifth baby . . . your last labour was induced and you had a forceps delivery . . . you have had a previous Caesarean section."

At the first antenatal visit the doctor may refer to a "risk score" in order to decide which category of care is appropriate for you: ordinary doctor/midwife or doctor/nurse care, specialized care under the direction of obstetricians, or highly specialized and intensive care involving expert teams. You may have little choice about this. Women are labelled high or low risk either on the basis of a score like this, or simply because of the doctor's clinical hunches. With some risk scores as many as nine out of ten women turn out to be high risk.

Attaching labels to pregnant women in this way – even when done with discretion – is damaging. A woman assigned to a high-risk category will probably have interventions that make birth more complicated, and women who are aware that they are "at risk" lose confidence and become anxious. If everyone around you *expects* things to go wrong, you begin to believe that they will – and they may well do so.

Often a woman is categorized as high or low risk without reference to the conditions of her everyday life. Such things as poor housing, bad conditions in the workplace, little money for food, a violent partner, social isolation, unemployment, or family problems are social conditions which are at the roots of perinatal mortality (baby deaths) and morbidity (illness).

Assigning all black women to an "at risk" category is racially discriminatory. There are wide variations in the life-styles, economic circumstances, and the education of black women. Asian women who live in one area of London have no more baby deaths than the general population, whereas those in Bradford, in the North of England, are much more likely to suffer the death of a baby. It is not a matter of skin colour but of socio-economic conditions.

In terms of improving the care of individual women, exercises in risk prediction are, according to Iain Chalmers, an obstetrician who is Director of the National Perinatal Epidemiology Unit in Britain, "a complete waste of time".* Birth, like all other human activities, is never risk-free. Even in a prosperous area of the British Isles, for example, there is a 5 per cent chance that birth will be pre-term, a 2 in 5 chance that a baby born before 28 weeks will live, an overall chance of 1 in a 100 that a baby will die, and a 1

"People say, 'How brave you are, having your baby at home!' I don't feel brave at all! I think they're the brave ones, to go into hospital, and risk all the things that are done to you there."

in 50 chance that a full-term baby will have a handicap. One woman in 10,000 dies because of something to do with a pregnancy. And, depending on where you have your baby, there is a 1 in 200 or a 1 in 4 chance (as in many parts of the USA) that delivery will be by Caesarean section.

Most of the risk markers used are very poor predictors. Some doctors still believe, for example, that any woman with small feet must have a small pelvic outlet too, so women are asked what size shoes they wear, and those wearing size 3 are automatically categorized as high risk. Research reveals that this is ridiculous.*

"They just told me what they were going to do. They never asked what I wanted."

Women often feel trapped with care that is imposed on them, and that is very different from that which they would have chosen themselves. It would be far better if doctors studied individual women to evaluate what care is appropriate to them, taking into account each woman's views and requests.

To be able to make decisions about care and about the place of birth, you need to have full and accurate information about potential risks and then to decide yourself what to do. Some risk is acceptable. We may want to go on holiday, so we take a plane. We enjoy skiing or rock-climbing and accept the risk of a broken leg. The risks are worth it. If sailors worried about risk all the time, they would never go to sea.

We can also prepare to handle risks, taking sensible precautions against the most likely dangers, such as wearing a life-jacket on a sailing dinghy, or buckling on a safety belt in the car, and we can learn what to do in the event that risks mount.

UNRAVELLING THE STATISTICS

It is often claimed that, because far fewer mothers die around the time of birth than, say, 60 years ago when most women had their babies at home, hospital birth must be the cause of this decline in the maternal and perinatal mortality rates. But the fact that two things happen at the same time does not mean that one causes the other.

Nor should we compare statistics of home births in different historical periods. Many things change, including women's health, their access to contraceptives and abortion, and their socio-economic conditions. These things have a profound effect on perinatal mortality. As the standard of living rises, fewer babies die at birth in every country, whether or not home births are allowed, and whatever the obstetric practice is.

Unplanned births outside hospital are often included in the statistics for home births, and this gives a completely wrong impression of the comparative risks of home and hospital births. Women who have

Thoughts on "risk"
by Judith Dickson Luce*

word so small
            born a verb
            an "action word"

                as I learned in 4th grade
                    I risk
                        you risk
                            she risks
            even a noun something
                            I take
                            you take
                            she takes

in philosophy a description of what life is
    with its own rewards:
        I love and risk loss and pain
            I try and risk failure
                I trust and risk betrayal
                I live and risk death
but we've moved so far beyond philosophy
        to insurance – for anything and everything
            to machines
            to technology and control
                (not daring)

and computers spit out the risk we are "at"
    before we breathe
        before we take a first step
            that might lead us to fall
and the computers and the statisticians tell us
    it is healthier and safer
        and wiser not to take risks
            since we are "at risk"
    and they can reduce risk
        and with it our capacity
            for living
                and touching
                    and caring
        it's safer that way
            neater and more efficient
                and definitely more sterile
and what more can we ask of life?

Commentary by Tom Luce: *"It's very risky to be born since very few people who are born avoid dying (although many avoid living). If you are born there is a high statistical risk you might die."*

unplanned out-of-hospital births may be delivering long before the baby is ready for life, or teenagers hiding a pregnancy and delivering somewhere, anywhere, where they hope their parents will not find out about the baby, or women delivering in panic on the way to hospital, or those who have had no antenatal care at all – the very poor, mentally confused, severely depressed, or drug addicted.

Planned home birth is safe. In Australia, where home birth is on the increase, 3,400 planned home births were analysed by the National Perinatal Statistics Unit.* The perinatal mortality rate was as low as 5.9 per 1,000. Some of these women were "high risk" and 30.8 per cent were what doctors call "untried pelvises", because they were giving birth for the first time. The figures include 15 multiple births, breech deliveries, women who had previous Caesarean sections (one had had three Caesarean births) and women with previous stillbirths.

These mothers tended to be older than the national average. (One woman was 47.) In all, 8.6 per cent moved to hospital during labour, usually because things were taking a long time, and 2.4 per cent of babies were transferred to hospital either for observation or because they needed specialized care.

There was remarkably little obstetric intervention in these home births. The Caesarean section rate was 2.2 per cent and only 3.1 per cent had forceps delivery or vacuum extraction. Few women had episiotomies – 20.1 per cent compared with 39.9 per cent of women delivering in Australian hospitals altogether, and about twice as many hospital mothers required suturing, either for an episiotomy or a tear.

"If anything goes wrong in hospital, they say: 'How lucky that you were in hospital!' They don't realize that it's because of what was done in hospital that things may have gone badly."

Yet in most countries it is assumed by both doctors and the general public that birth outside hospital must be dangerous and, as perinatal mortality rates are dropping in all industrialized countries, it is believed that this must be because most women now have their babies in hospital.

In Britain Marjorie Tew was the first person to challenge the assumption that the rise in hospital births was directly responsible for the drop in deaths. She taught statistics in the Department of Community Health at Nottingham University Medical School and set her students the task of discovering all that they could about the maternal and perinatal mortality rates. She expected that the published data would confirm the view that hospital birth is safest, but was amazed to find "that maternal and fetal death rates for comparable groups were always higher in hospital than at home whether the predicted risk . . . was high or low."*

At first no medical journal would publish her findings, so she published elsewhere. Doctors often treated her with scorn and derision. Other statisticians sat on the fence or entered the fray brandishing questionable – Marjorie Tew called them "spurious" – statistics of their own. She was fired from her job but went on tenaciously with her work, funding it herself.*

It has come to be accepted by most women, as well as the vast majority of doctors, that hospital must be the safest place. In 1980 the Social Services Committee of the House of Commons recommended that more women should be delivered in large units and home birth "phased out further".* In its report it produced a graph showing that more babies died at home than in hospital. Hidden in those statistics was the fact that *unplanned* out-of-hospital births accounted for the increase in deaths.* Though the Social Services Committee recommended that isolated GP (general practitioner) units should be closed down and that women should have their babies in large regional centres, their statistics actually showed that in these small hospitals birth was very safe. The committee seems to have come to its conclusions without understanding its own statistics.

Statistics resulting from 1958 and 1970 perinatal surveys in Britain*				
Place	*Percentage of births*		*Perinatal mortality rate per 1,000 births*	
	1958	*1970*	*1958*	*1970*
Hospital	49	66	50.1	27.8
General practitioner unit	12	19	20.3	6.1
Home	36	12	19.8	4.3

Statistics of perinatal mortality rates according to risk score of mother*		
Perinatal mortality rate per 1,000 births		
Risk	Hospital	General practitioner unit/home
Very low	8.0	3.9
Low	17.9	5.2
Moderate	32.2	3.8
High	53.2	15.5
Very high	162.6	133.3
Number of births	11,000	5,200

As more and more women went into hospitals staffed by specialist obstetric teams, the majority of them *low risk* who would have previously given birth in a small GP unit or at home, the number of babies dying in these hospitals went *up*.* Marjorie Tew then analysed the statistics produced by the British Birth Survey of 1970* and, using the risk scores employed by the survey's researchers, showed that, except for the women at the very greatest risk, birth was safer at home or in a GP unit than in hospital.*

As fewer and fewer women had home births or births in isolated GP units in Britain, it became more difficult to compare the results of births in these places with those in large hospitals. So Marjorie Tew turned her attention to the Netherlands, where 38 per cent of babies are still born at home, and analysed the perinatal mortality statistics there.

Perinatal mortality rate in the Netherlands 1986*		
	Hospital	*Home*
Number of births	119,037	66,536
Number of deaths	1,653	149
Perinatal mortality rate per 1,000	13.9	2.2

In the Netherlands women having babies at home may be cared for either by a midwife or a general practitioner, and in hospital by midwives or doctors. If you look at baby deaths both in terms of *where* the birth took place and of *who attended* the births, some astonishing statistics emerge.

The Netherlands 1986 Perinatal mortality rate by birth attendant and place*			
Attendant	*Place*	*Number of births*	*Perinatal mortality rate per 1,000 births*
Obstetrician	Hospital	83,351	18.9
GP	Home	21,653	4.5
Midwives	Hospital	34,874	2.1
Midwives	Home	44,676	1.0

Care given by a midwife at home is safer than care from midwives in hospital, and home birth with a midwife is safest of all.

For mothers having their first babies, birth at home with a midwife also proves to be safer than birth with an obstetrician.

First births in the Netherlands 1986*		
	Obstetrician in hospital	*Midwife at home*
Number of births	41,861	15,031
Perinatal mortality rate per 1,000	20.2	1.5

The proportion of women at high risk who have their babies in hospital cannot explain this enormous difference in perinatal mortality. But what about babies born pre-term? Here is Marjorie Tew's analysis of deaths of babies born at under 36 weeks, according to who attended the birth:

Pre-term babies*		
Pre-term babies	*Under obstetric care*	*Under midwife care*
Proportion of all births less than 37 weeks	7.6	1.8
Perinatal mortality rate per 1,000	85.7	30.1

These statistics should be interpreted with caution because obstetricians may have attended a larger proportion of *very* pre-term births, which would be at higher risk. Even so, this is a huge difference.

Marjorie Tew concludes that "complications are more likely to occur in hospital because of, not in spite of, high-tech intervention . . . The threat of home birth is not a threat to mother and baby but a threat to the healthy survival of obstetric and medical professions."*

LOOKING AT THE RISKS

Smoking
If you smoke, the single most important thing you can do to reduce risk to yourself and your baby is to stop smoking before you get pregnant or in the first half of the pregnancy, or at least to cut it down below ten cigarettes a

day. Many midwives in the USA and Canada will not accept home birth clients who smoke during pregnancy, because of the associated risks.

Nicotine constricts blood vessels so that the flow of blood through the placenta is slower, and this can lead to intra-uterine growth retardation (IUGR). Carbon monoxide and thiocynate in cigarette smoke also reduce the baby's growth. Smokers are more at risk of miscarriage, of having pre-term babies, and of haemorrhage from the placenta. A woman who smokes *and* drinks alcohol takes even greater risks.

Alcohol

In North America the fetal alcohol syndrome is the most usual teratogenic cause (that is, damage caused while the baby is in the uterus) of mental handicap. This may occur when a woman drinks around eight glasses of wine or four pints of beer a day. You don't have to drink this much, however, to make it more likely that a baby will be born with low birth weight. There is some evidence that if you drink more than ten glasses of wine a week the baby does not grow so well in the uterus.*

Your weight

If you are very underweight or overweight, this may affect your pregnancy and labour too. If you are very underweight, there is a chance that the baby will not be well nourished. If you are very fat, you are more likely to have raised blood pressure and to develop pregnancy diabetes, both of which will lead to your being advised not to give birth at home.* Being fat means that you are also more likely to develop a urinary infection or to have a blood clot during pregnancy. But if you are healthy, there is no added risk to the baby; healthy overweight women give birth to healthy babies.* The customary practice of being weighed regularly in pregnancy, and all the worry that results, is worse than useless. The height of the fundus (the top of the uterus) is a far more important gauge of the baby's growth.

If you want home birth, it helps to be within a normal weight range. You and your caregivers are likely to feel happier about it. But, if you are overweight, never go on a crash diet during pregnancy. This is bad for both you and your baby. All you need do is to cut down on fat and sugar and foods containing these.

Your blood pressure

It is quite natural for blood pressure to rise a little at the very end of pregnancy, and this does not make birth any less safe.* But, if your blood pressure is up and at the same time protein (albumen) appears in your urine and your skin becomes puffy with retained fluid, you have pre-eclampsia and, unless it is very mild, will usually be advised to have your baby in hospital, because the placenta may not be functioning well.

If your blood pressure is rising, look at ways in which you can cut down stress and take life easier. Pamper yourself and, if you possibly can, go to bed and ask other people to shop, cook, and clean. Listen to music, read, practise your relaxation, and get someone you love to massage you with a soporific aromatherapy oil. If you already have other children, this is very difficult to do unless there are other people close to you who can take over the children. You can always cuddle up with a toddler in bed, with picture books, television, and some new playthings, but two-year-olds are not the most restful little people to have around, and the therapy for your high blood pressure will have to be a compromise between care for yourself and the joys and responsibilities of mothering. But, however you work it out, getting more rest gives you the best chance of being healthy at the end of the pregnancy, and still being able to have your baby at home. If this is your first baby, remember that once the baby is born you will never have the opportunity to lie around luxuriously like this again, so enjoy it!

You are over 35

If you are having your first baby over the age of 35, or with some doctors even over 30, you are considered an "elderly primigravida", at greater risk of what obstetricians sometimes call "poor obstetric performance". Some even describe older mothers as "obstetrically senescent" or "geriatric".*

Nowadays women having their first baby in their thirties have not necessarily had a long history of fertility problems – something that is associated with increased risk – but have delayed motherhood because of their professional careers or until they felt ready to have a child. Their education and socio-economic conditions mean that they are in a low-risk group compared with, say, those teenagers who become pregnant accidentally or because they want someone to love. The perinatal mortality rate for these older mothers is no higher than that for younger mothers.*

What is different is the amount of obstetric intervention that older mothers receive in hospital. In one London hospital women over 35 are more than twice as likely to have labour augmented with oxytocin (53 per cent compared with 20 per cent of under-35s), to have an episiotomy (74 per cent compared with 38 per cent), to be delivered by forceps (35 per cent compared with 25 per cent) or to have a Caesarean section (28 per cent compared with 13 per cent).* The researchers who established these figures thought that the high rate of Caesarean section may have occurred because more older mothers receive continuous electronic monitoring, and suggested that anxiety on the part of obstetricians may contribute to the aggressive management of labour with older mothers. One way of avoiding this, which is a valid option if you have a healthy pregnancy and if there are no special contra-indications, is to have your baby in a birth centre or GP unit or at home.

A breech baby

Three or four babies in every 100 are born bottom first.* Problems can arise because, although the baby's body may slip through easily, the head may get caught inside the mother's body, and delay at delivery can result in oxygen deprivation.

In some countries Caesarean sections are performed for most breech births, on the grounds that it is better to be safe than sorry. In Sweden, for example, nine out of ten breech babies are sections. Compare this with Norway, where only four or five are sections. If you live in a country where you know that if you have your baby in hospital you are more or less bound to have a Caesarean, then you may feel that a home or birth centre birth is an attractive alternative, as long as you can arrange for skilled and experienced care. On the other hand, you may find that your caregivers are very reluctant to take on the extra risk of a breech birth. To give you the best care at home, it is important that your midwife and/or doctor feel confident about their roles and about you.

When interpreting statistics, bear in mind that many breech babies – more than 30 per cent – are born like this because they are pre-term (not yet 37 weeks). It is only as a baby becomes heavier that it tips head-down. If you go to term and have a breech baby, there is not the added risk associated with pre-term babies.

Babies who are breech in late pregnancy often somersault and are head-down by the time labour starts. About 14 per cent are breech at 32 weeks,* and there is a three in five chance of them turning after that time, and still at 36 weeks a one in four chance,* though this is less likely if the baby's legs are extended, because legs splint the body, making it harder for the baby to roll over. Some babies even kick themselves round once labour has actually started, provided that they have enough space.

So, if you are planning a home birth, you need not be steam-rollered in the last weeks of pregnancy into changing the birthplace. It is reasonable to delay making a final decision until you are at term.

A previous pre-term baby

If you have had a baby before who was born pre-term, there is an increased possibility that this will happen again, but you still have an 83 per cent chance of going to full term. Even if you have had two pre-term births, there is still a 72 per cent chance that this will not recur.*

A previous Caesarean section

If you have had a previous Caesarean section, you will certainly be advised by doctors to have your next baby and all other babies in hospital. Many obstetricians in North America do repeat Caesarean sections even when the same problems do not recur in another labour. This is one reason why the Caesarean section rate has multiplied five times in the last 20 years.

British obstetricians adopt a different approach. They allow a "trial" of labour. This is really a trial of the scar, with everything ready for Caesarean section in case it splits open. That means a hospital birth of course.

Rupture of the uterus occurs extremely rarely. In a series of 110,000 births following previous Caesarean section there were 13 ruptures.*

Most of the papers in medical journals on which doctors base their policies warn against rupture following the old-fashioned "classical" Caesarean section, when the incision in the uterus is vertical. Nowadays most incisions are horizontal, in the lower segment of the uterus, just about at the level of the top of a bikini.

The risks of rupture are much reduced when a horizontal, lower-segment incision has been made and, even when the scar does not stand up to the strain, it does not pop open, but one edge unpeels slightly.

It is hard to know how to advise a woman who has had a Caesarean section and who wants a home birth. There are additional risks in having a baby outside hospital, but there are also risks with unnecessary and harmful interventions that occur in many hospitals, and it may be that the previous Caesarean section was the result of intervention. Choosing birth outside hospital is for many women the only way of avoiding these risks.

MEDICAL CONDITIONS

Sometimes pregnant women are told by doctors that, if they suffer from certain illnesses, such as diabetes, they must give birth in hospital. They can make a strong case for diabetic mothers because, with all that sugar in the blood, babies often grow very large. In the past babies of diabetic mothers often had breathing problems. But, now that there is good insulin control during pregnancy, fewer than 2 in 100 have breathing problems.*

If you have an illness that gets worse when you are under stress, however, home may be the best place for you if you feel more secure and confident there. With asthma, for example, there is no increased risk to the baby, and a good case for having a baby at home.* With multiple sclerosis, home may be the ideal place too.*

You are Rhesus negative
Your blood is tested for the Rhesus factor in early pregnancy. If you are Rhesus negative and the baby's father is Rhesus positive, you have further tests later in pregnancy to find out whether you are developing antibodies to a Rhesus positive baby. This is extremely unlikely to happen if it is your first baby and if you have not had a previous miscarriage, but you should know that the risk increases if anything is done that causes bleeding in pregnancy, such as chorionic villus sampling, amniocentesis, and fetoscopy.

Interventions during labour and at delivery can also cause leaking of the baby's blood into your own and result in sensitization in the next pregnancy. These include fixing a scalp clip to the baby's head to monitor the heart-rate, forceps delivery or Caesarean section, accidental tearing of the cord if it is pulled in an attempt to deliver the placenta, and manual removal of the placenta. So childbirth without unnecessary intervention is the safest course of action, which may mean that birth at home or in a birth centre or GP unit is best.

The discovery of gamma-globulin in the 60s, and its regular use now when a Rhesus negative woman is likely to be bearing a Rhesus positive baby, has saved many lives. You may be given injections of anti-D immunoglobulin during pregnancy, at the birth, or within five days of the birth of a Rhesus positive baby to avoid sensitization in the next pregnancy, and will be screened regularly during subsequent pregnancies.

Fewer than 1 baby in 1,000 dies today from problems associated with Rhesus incompatibility. Provided that you do not develop antibodies during pregnancy, your baby and you are not at increased risk. You should be able to choose the place where you would like to have your baby.

THE RISKS OF HOME BIRTH

The following risks are often cited for birth at home and in a place where only low technology is available:

☐ *A long labour with slow dilatation of the cervix.*
A long labour is tiring but, unless other problems develop, is not in itself

dangerous, although labours that last more than 48 hours in hospital often lead to forceps delivery, vacuum extraction, or Caesarean section, which may themselves introduce risk. There is no relation between long labour (over 24 hours) and mental handicap in babies.*

☐ *Prolapsed cord.*
Prolapsed cord occurs when the membranes rupture and the presenting part of the baby – head or buttocks – is high, so that there is space for the cord to drop down. Pressure on the cord can reduce the blood flow to the baby and deprive it of oxygen. The cord cannot drop down when the head is engaged and lying over the cervix. This is one reason why a pregnant woman has antenatal care, and why her caregivers palpate her abdomen and find out the position of the baby every week at the end of pregnancy.

☐ *Cephalo-pelvic disproportion, where the baby's head is too big to pass through the mother's pelvis.*
Cephalo-pelvic disproportion (CPD) is often misdiagnosed simply because labour is long, and Caesarean section is performed for that reason. When it is obvious that a baby cannot pass through the mother's pelvis she should go to hospital. This is not a sudden emergency. It is a decision made after much discussion when it is clear that no progress is being made.

☐ *A long second stage.*
A long second stage is tiring but not in itself dangerous.

☐ *Shoulder dystocia with a big baby, where the head emerges, but then the shoulders are stuck.*
When shoulders get stuck, they can be released if the mother turns on to all-fours, she is delivered from behind and, if the shoulders are very large, an episiotomy is made.

☐ *Breathing difficulties at birth.*
Babies are most likely to have breathing difficulties when their mothers have had pain-killing drugs in labour, including pethidine, sedatives, tranquillizers, and epidural anaesthesia. A woman having a baby at home often has no drugs at all or, if she chooses to have them, has only a very small dose. Simple ways of resuscitating a baby – clearing the airways, giving oxygen and massage – can be used at home.

☐ *Postpartum haemorrhage.*
Postpartum haemorrhage is most likely to occur when there has been obstetric intervention in birth or attempts have been made to pull the placenta out before it has completely separated from the uterine wall. If

"Midwives carry oxygen to give a baby if necessary, but the doctors I saw didn't realize that. I want a home birth because I am anxious to avoid my delivery becoming as medicalized as those I witnessed during my training."
A general practitioner having her first baby

50

there is bleeding, artificial oxytocin in the form of syntometrine can be given by injection to make the uterus contract firmly, and it is simple to do this at home.

Handling the risks of home birth

If you want to have your baby at home, it makes sense to:

☐ Find a good midwife. She should be skilled, confident, and relaxed in working in an out-of-hospital setting.

☐ Get all the information you can about how to help yourself in childbirth. Learn the art of meeting contractions with relaxation, breathing, and focused concentration, and find out how a variety of positions and movements can assist descent and rotation of the baby. Approach birth free from fear, self-assured, and positive.

☐ Ensure that there is more than one birth attendant and that your caregivers work well together: a midwife needs her own support. Immediately after the birth you and the baby may need attention at the same time.

☐ Ensure that you have access to a telephone and specialized care if you or the baby needs it. You can either use your own transport to get to hospital, or there may be a team from hospital (the obstetric flying squad) which will come to you if you have a retained placenta or other problem.

☐ Make sure that simple equipment and medications are available that can be used in an out-of-hospital setting: for example, a Pinard's stethoscope or, better still, a sonic aid; drugs to make the uterus contract after the baby is born if you bleed a good deal; some simple methods of pain relief, such as hot compresses, a bath or shower; and oxygen.

☐ Make certain that your home is reasonably clean, comfortable, and convenient for giving birth, with hot and cold water, and a means of heating in cold weather and air cooling in hot weather.

The baby's safety

Whenever a woman decides to have a home birth, there are people who suggest that either the baby might die from neglect because it is not born in a hospital setting, or that it might be mentally damaged from lack of oxygen. The perinatal mortality rate for planned home births is very low indeed – 3 to 4 per 1,000 compared with 9 to 10 per 1,000 births as a whole. Moreover two of these three or four deaths are unavoidable wherever the baby is born, because the baby is extremely pre-term or suffers a congenital handicap that is incompatible with life. All that birth in a high-tech hospital might do is delay death by a few days or weeks.

Ninety-two per cent of all mental handicap in babies occurs *before* labour, either as the result of congenital malformation (around 63 per cent) or of events and processes that occurred during pregnancy, such as intra-uterine growth retardation (8 per cent), infections such as rubella (6 per cent), or accidents such as lead poisoning. The damage occurred long before labour started.*

In a hospital with an intensive care unit a severely handicapped baby is taken immediately for all life-saving procedures that are available to be employed. Being in hospital may make the difference between death and survival with a major handicap. Some women choose home birth because they would not want vigorous and extraordinary methods to be used to save the life of a damaged baby. Others choose hospital because they want the baby to have every chance of life, however severe the handicap.

"Working in an intensive care unit, I see many babies being kept alive who I think should have been allowed to die in peace. That's one reason why I've decided on a home birth."

It is an enormous responsibility to bring a baby into the world, and it starts long before the baby is in your arms. There are doctors who accuse women having home birth of "child abuse", and who would even like to prosecute them. They see it as a choice only a selfish woman would make, and see themselves as the saviours of babies, rescuing them from their egotistical, hysterical mothers. Yet your informed decision to give birth at home or in a birth centre or small GP unit may be one way in which you accept deep personal responsibility for your baby. There is no reason to think that if you have a planned birth outside hospital you are risking your baby's life or intelligence. It can be a choice that you make not only for your own, but for your baby's sake.

CHARLOTTE'S HOME BIRTH

Charlotte is a schoolteacher, and this is her third baby.

She had a show, but for the following 48 hours had contractions only when she moved around.

To get labour going she and her birth companion, Janet, went for a long walk in nearby woods the next afternoon. But regular contractions, five minutes apart, did not start till late evening. She called her midwife at 11 p.m., who examined her and said, "You're not at all dilated." So she went to bed. At 4.30 a.m. powerful contractions woke her. "But because someone in authority had told me I was not dilating, I couldn't take them seriously. It was only at 7.15 a.m., when I tried to read the children their third morning story, that I thought, 'I must do something about this!'" Suddenly it was as if the labour jumped two gears. She crouched on the floor, feeling pulled down by gravity, and swayed, rocked, and groaned. "I have never felt anything so strong." The two midwives turned up at 8.30 a.m. By then she was kneeling with her arms on the bed. One of them examined her: "I had a vision of jumping out of the window if I was not dilating." But she was fully dilated. "I knew exactly what I was doing. I hardly had to push at all. It wasn't painful, and the baby slipped out in a calm, very controlled way at 8.40 a.m. It was wonderful!"

In hospital babies are weighed on a balance scale. They usually hate this, flail around and cry. At home, a midwife often uses a spring scale, with the baby nestled in soft cloth suspended from it. Firmly cradled like this, a baby may not cry at all.

"I couldn't believe that here was a beautiful, healthy baby. I was completely bowled over! I laughed. There was a huge welling up of happiness. I feel I have been celebrating ever since – a bubbly feeling, like the fizz in champagne."

"Janet made me feel cherished. Her support during labour was important because I knew that she would not collude with doctors. Here was an ally. If I couldn't articulate what I wanted, she could articulate for me. She cherished me afterwards, too. She 'happened to be passing – with a meal' and asked, 'Can I share it with you?' I spent a week surrounded by women to whom I was close. They camped out here, and we had picnics."

"Imogen is Janet's baby as well as mine. We were on the same wavelength. When you share birth with another woman, you know that she understands with a great deal more clarity than a man what you are feeling or thinking. There was something about being surrounded by women, all giving loving support, that was very comforting. It felt secure, warm, and very strong. It was something that we all did together."

Louise is five and William three-and-a-half. They came in immediately after the baby slipped out, and were fascinated by her. Louise went to school next day "just shining, from top to toe".

"It made the birth special to have the children there so quickly after, and to be able to share their wonder. I needed them. I couldn't have borne to be parted from them. And it was wonderful to sleep afterwards in a big bed with all my children."

Charlotte freshened up in a warm bath, with the baby nestled close to her.

Arranging a Birth Without Hospital

Depending on where you live, you may have the choice between giving birth in an alternative birth centre (ABC), linked with or completely separate from a hospital, in a small GP unit, in an independent midwife-staffed clinic where the focus is on supporting physiological birth rather than obstetrics, or at home. It is worth exploring your options.

THE ALTERNATIVE BIRTH CENTRE: HOME FROM HOME?

A birth centre is a maternity unit which, at least ideally, provides exclusively low-technology care, where there is a homely atmosphere, and from which women return home in a matter of hours after giving birth. In the United States, where the first birth centre was established in New York in 1975, ABCs have mushroomed over the last ten years. Caregivers are for the most part nurse–midwives or nurses working with an obstetrician, though in some centres there are midwives with no nursing background.

A birth centre may be free-standing and separate from a hospital, in hospital grounds, or inside a hospital building. The important thing about it is that it should have a distinct atmosphere of its own and *its special staff*. The policy of the Family Health Program Birth Center in Salt Lake City, for example, is "to provide safe maternity care to low-risk families, in a home-like, out-of-hospital setting," and achieve "parental satisfaction through a highly educational, personalized form of care, which encourages intra-family contact and participation in the management . . . of childbearing . . . Childbirth is a peak life experience and is viewed as a healthy process. Confidence in the physiologic function of the body to cope with childbirth is promoted in all aspects of care." Health care providers are educators and resource people to enable women themselves to take on the responsibility for their own health. A birth centre that is simply a set of rooms decorated to look attractive alongside other rooms in the delivery suite, and that does not have its own staff, is one in name only. Many hospitals have introduced birth rooms with paintings on the walls, flowered wallpaper, hanging plants, and rocking chairs, in which there is no special philosophy of care that arises from a holistic approach to childbirth, and where as much obstetric intervention takes place as in the more clinical-looking rooms along the corridor.

In an alternative birth centre worthy of the name, there is no induction and no augmentation of labour with oxytocin, no electronic fetal monitoring except for Doppler ultrasound – the sonic aid – there are no drugs for pain relief, except local analgesia to suture tears in the perineum, very few episiotomies, and no operative deliveries. In many the only equipment is oxygen, and catheters for clearing a baby's airways when they are blocked.

In the Garden of Life Birth Center in Dearborn, Michigan, where the focus is on cultural sensitivity to the needs of the Muslim, Italian, Hispanic, Polish, and Anglo parents using the centre, the sole machinery is a coffee-maker. Staff wear ordinary clothing, not uniforms. Women can move around in labour and adopt any position they like for birth. Childbirth education is an integral part of the programme, and other members of the family can be present at the birth. The bed is king-sized, low, and comfortable, so that mother, father, and new baby can cuddle together.

ABCs tend to have very strict rules as to who may use them. Some, such as the New York Maternity Childbearing Center, screen out half of the women who apply to use them. This may be partly because of legal or insurance restrictions, partly because many ABCs are administered or funded by a health authority or hospital. Women expecting twins, those with pre-eclampsia or diabetes, or those who develop problems during pregnancy – suspected fetal growth retardation, for instance – are usually excluded from giving birth in these centres.

Midwives and nurses working independently in birth centres and small clinics, even in countries where midwifery is already a strong profession, as in Sweden, find a satisfying new role and exciting relationship with the families they are helping. In the ABC unit at Sodersjkuhuset, Stockholm, for example, it is a midwife, not a doctor, who makes the decision as to whether labour is deviating from the normal and who then refers a woman to obstetric care in the same building. In this ABC such a referral happens with one woman in ten during pregnancy. In the early days a further 30 per cent were moved during labour, often for oxytocin stimulation of the uterus because their waters had broken and there were no contractions, or labour was slow, but as midwives became more confident this very high percentage of transfers was halved in the first six months. In most American ABCs between 7 and 16 per cent of women are switched to regular obstetric care because they require drugs for pain relief, have slow labours, or there is failure to progress. You will need to bear this in mind if you decide you would like to give birth in an ABC.

Choosing a good birth centre

In a good birth centre you can expect architecture on a human scale and attractive interior design, with such things as comfortable furniture, photographs of the midwives with their names on the notice board, and many photographs of mothers with their new babies, pictures, sculptures, mobiles, and other representations of birth and womb-ripeness. Rooms are often carpeted, lighting can be dimmed, there are curtains at the windows, beanbags and relaxation chairs, maybe a patchwork quilt, and a wooden crib or muslin-hung cot. You have your own bathroom with a large bath tub, perhaps a jacuzzi, and a powerful shower for back massage. There may be a birth pool in which you can labour and give birth if you wish. The

"I saw my baby's head crowning and she was placed on my tummy. No tubes were forced down her throat. She was born amid laughter and joy, shared by all. Our second child is almost due and will be born in the same peaceful, gentle atmosphere of Boothville."

"I enjoyed being looked after as a Special Mum, as everyone was treated there, and I treasure the warmth and fun that was shared with those midwives and doctors."

whole atmosphere is relaxing and non-clinical, offering a space in which you and your partner can be private, locking the door when you want to. No shining instruments are in evidence, though there may be some tucked behind the curtain. You can bring in things you would like to have around you and wear your own clothes, not institutional garb.

The kitchen is often located centrally in the building and is a gathering-place for expectant parents, midwives, and new parents as they talk over cups of tea. In the Stockholm ABC parents have their own fridge and make meals when they want them. No one serves up meals at set times. The father or mother, or perhaps a grandparent, makes a snack whenever they wish. In a very different birth centre in El Paso, Texas, the kitchen is also the heart of the centre – but, in contrast to the style of the modern white-wood Swedish kitchen with its bundles of dried rosebuds, this is a Mexican kitchen, familiar and comforting for the mothers who walk across the border in labour to give birth in the United States, and hope that in this way their babies may become American citizens. Instead of Swedish cheese and shortbread cookies, you sniff the odours of Mexican dishes based on black beans and peppers.

Antenatal care in birth centres is given by the midwives or nurses, who may be available for as long as two hours at a time to talk through emotional aspects of the birth experience, and who do not limit care to doing tests. In fact in some birth centres you are shown how to test your urine and check your own blood pressure at home.

"I was told that every first-time mother had Demerol [pethidine]. It wasn't a question of whether she thought she needed it."

But there are many phoney birth centres. As health care entrepreneurs and hospital administrators have caught on to the ABC as a major marketing opportunity, a venture that could make their hospital more competitive with others, the original concept has been diluted. Those who own a birth centre – business people, doctors, a health authority, hospital, or whatever – control how it is run and everything that happens in it. If a birth centre is not run by the midwives who work in it, you should be particularly careful about examining all the pros and cons. Just because a maternity unit is called an ABC, do not assume that care is woman-centred. In US birth centres as a whole, 15 per cent of women have intravenous infusions and 9 per cent enemas, though only 8 per cent have episiotomies. The typical Californian centre is physician-owned in a commercial building, with a couple of birth rooms, and births are attended by the obstetricians. Californian physician-owned insurance companies will not usually provide malpractice cover for ABCs unless they are on hospital grounds, and only obstetricians can do deliveries. Malpractice insurance is too high for most family practitioners to risk working in an ABC, and nurse–midwives have

"There is a time-limit on labour, and then they shove you in a hospital. This hospital has a 30 per cent Caesarean section rate."

great difficulty in obtaining insurance cover to work in birth centres unless they are supervised by an obstetrician.

In the United States non-profit institutions staffed by nurse–midwives or registered midwives with back-up from a sympathetic obstetrician are giving way to hundreds of profit centres, and, as in Australia and increasingly in Europe, hospitals offer ABCs or birth rooms as a cosmetic exercise to attract more customers. Yet the non-profit birth centres that can still be found often provide most value for money: offering more childbirth education, more prenatal care, more classes for siblings, and more home visits after the birth.

Along with the increase in physician-operated centres, some American obstetricians have equipped their offices to do out-of-hospital births, both in response to consumer demand and to make a fast buck. Procedures used may include paracervical blocks (pain-killing injections around the cervix), electronic fetal monitoring, ultrasound, induction and augmentation of labour, vacuum extraction, forceps, and even, in at least one ABC, Caesarean section.

"It's run by a cosmetic surgeon, with an obstetrician on call. He has an office downstairs where he does the cosmetic surgery."

As obstetricians take over the birth centre movement, they also transfer their concept of birth as a medical event, and with it increasing dependence on technology.

Questions to ask

When enquiring about a particular birth centre, you may want to ask the following questions:

☐ What is your transfer rate during pregnancy? (This will enable you to estimate what your chances are of actually having your baby in the birth centre.)

☐ What is your transfer rate during labour? (A rate of between 7 and 12 per cent is reasonable.)

☐ Do you ever induce labour with oxytocin and/or amniotomy?

☐ Is electronic fetal monitoring used? (Doppler ultrasound, in the form of a hand-held sonic aid, for intermittent monitoring is acceptable. Scalp clips and abdominal belts are not.)

☐ Is intravenous glucose given?

☐ Are pain-relieving drugs used?

☐ Do you provide epidural anaesthesia?

☐ Is labour ever augmented with oxytocin?

☐ Is there a time limit on the second stage?

☐ What percentage of women have episiotomies? (It should be less than 10 per cent.)

☐ Do you ever do forceps delivery or vacuum extraction?

The answers to these questions may make you want to ask more. If any of these procedures are used, it will help to know if they are employed more or less routinely or rarely, so you may wish to ask for percentages of different interventions in the previous year.

Other questions concern your freedom to do whatever you feel like doing at the time:

☐ Can I walk around during labour?

☐ Can I deliver on the floor if I wish?

☐ Do women ever give birth standing up?

☐ How do you help a woman with backache labour?

☐ Can I get in the bath or shower during labour?

☐ What do you do when dilatation is slow?

☐ Is it possible for my other children to be present?

☐ May I eat and drink during labour if I want to?

☐ Will there be a midwife or nurse with me all the time through the late first stage?

☐ Do you have a birth pool that I can use?

The answers will give you an idea of the quality of care, but your spontaneous feelings are also a good guide. Your intuitive reactions about whether this is the place in which you would like to give birth are important. You need to feel relaxed, confident, secure, and among friends.

Birth centres have proved themselves safe, and in many of them few invasive, uncomfortable, restrictive procedures are used during birth. In the United States a national study of 11,814 women admitted to 84 free-standing birth centres revealed that the perinatal mortality rate was as low as 1.3 per 1,000 births* compared with 8 per 1,000 for all hospital births.*

In New York outcomes for low-risk mothers booked at the Maternity Center's Childbearing Center were compared with those for low-risk mothers at a large teaching hospital, Mount Sinai.* Women in hospital were more likely to have labour induced, and augmentation of labour occurred six times as frequently. Amniotomy more than two hours before the birth was more common, electronic fetal monitoring was used five times as often, four times as many women laboured with intravenous drips set up, more than double the number had drugs for pain relief, and there were eleven times as many epidurals. Women in the birth centre had noticeably longer second stages: over 80 per cent had second stages lasting more than two hours, compared with fewer than 19 per cent in the hospital. The incidence of thick meconium staining was three times greater for women in the hospital. (When some of the contents of the baby's bowel appear like this during labour, it can be a sign that the baby is over-stressed.) Women in the birth centre were four times as likely to have an intact perineum: that is, no tear and no episiotomy. Judging by live, healthy babies, birth was just as safe in the Childbearing Center as at this prestigious hospital, but with far less intervention and in a pleasanter environment.

In hospitals, even those advocating "family-centred" care, intervention rates are much higher. Research in Australian hospitals reveals that those with flexible policies aiming for sensitivity to parents' wishes still have high rates of induction of labour, oxytocin use, and operative deliveries.*

In birth centres or birth rooms that are an integral part of a hospital the orientation towards treating patients as high risk and using all techniques available spills over to low-risk women across the corridor. This takes place even though the benefits are marginal or non-existent and the interventions are sometimes harmful. In a Canadian hospital, for example, as many as 63 per cent of first-time mothers and 19 per cent of those who had already had babies were transferred from the birth room to the conventional hospital setting.* Clearly, if you are choosing a birth centre linked to a hospital, it is essential that it has its own staff and that they are confident and skilled enough to give continuing, low-technology care.

GP UNITS AND MIDWIFE CLINICS – SMALL IS BEAUTIFUL?

General practitioner units, sometimes isolated, such as exist in the UK and other European countries, and in Australia and New Zealand, grew out of cottage hospitals serving the community. Although the beds are "GP beds", most care is by midwives: the GP may not even turn up for the birth.

These small units are often homely and welcoming. Women like them because they already know the midwives and doctor, mothers and babies are kept together after birth as a matter of course, and they are near home. It is usually not possible to have an epidural or Caesarean section in a small unit like this, and a baby who needs special care must be moved to a larger hospital where there are intensive care facilities. Some of these units are quite old-fashioned, but many have kept the best of the old and incorporated active childbirth and gentle birth into their practice. The emphasis is usually on as little intervention as possible during birth and on a close, supportive relationship between the midwife and her client.

Isolated GP units have a good safety record. In the British Births 1970 survey, unpublished data – later made available to Marjorie Tew – revealed that the perinatal mortality rate for moderately high-risk women was more than ten times higher in obstetric hospitals than in isolated GP units, and even for high-risk women it was more than four times higher. For low-risk women it was 11 times higher. Only for very low-risk women was there not much difference, and even for them the perinatal mortality rate was higher by two-thirds.* This is true in other countries as well. In New Zealand, for example, babies of normal birth weight are more likely to die in large, high-tech hospitals than in small maternity units.*

If you are considering a GP unit, visit it first and ask the same questions that you might ask of a birth centre (see page 61), including the rate of transfer. You will probably have a one-to-one relationship with the midwife because she is attached to your GP's practice, the usual situation in Britain, and so you will be able to ask her how she avoids episiotomies, what she recommends if a woman has a slow, backache labour, how she feels about water birth, and so on. With a good midwife this type of dialogue is a vital part of the relationship between you. Midwives create the flavour of a GP unit. In some areas they are attached to the GP unit rather than to GP practices, so you may not meet them unless you go to the unit.

Protocols for running GP units are usually strict. You won't find high-tech gadgets sneaked in or interventionist obstetric techniques employed, although you may find that an amniotomy is done, or that there is an older midwife who likes her patients to have an enema. But it is more likely that you will find midwives who are keen for you to walk about during labour or soak in a bath, and who know how to help you have a physiological rather than a managed birth.

You may have the option of a small maternity unit that is staffed and run by midwives, although few such clinics exist. They are very similar to those GP units that are separate from large hospitals, and the atmosphere is warm,

"Everything was warm, friendly, and fuss-free. My husband was tired after a long flight, and as I was walking about and leaning on Sue, my midwife, when I had a contraction, and was in and out of the bath, she tucked him up in the bed for a snooze whilst we got on with it. Then, when contractions were coming every two minutes, she woke him up with a cup of tea so that he didn't miss anything. She showed him how to rub my back and we made a great team!"

friendly and relaxed. There is usually a good system of obstetric back-up combined with personal care from midwives whom you get to know before the birth.

Unfortunately, in most industrialized countries in Europe, North America, and Australia governments are closing down small hospitals and outlying GP units – in spite of a great deal of protest from consumers – on the grounds of safety, "rationalization", and economics. They are concentrating care in large regional centres with high-tech facilities, great gleaming edifices of steel and glass. With regionalization of care, women have to travel long distances to antenatal clinics and once they have started labour. Moreover care in these hospitals is focused on pathology, and tends to be less flexible and more impersonal than in small hospitals. There is often severe overcrowding in antenatal clinics, with long waiting times, and women are herded through them like cattle. Authoritarian attitudes set administrative convenience before the needs of the women for whom the service is supposed to exist.*

Many GP units even the most old-fashioned ones, have, at least potentially, the qualities of a good birth centre and offer a similar relaxed kind of care. Without either of these options, women are forced into standard hospital care, with its high intervention rates, unless they decide on home birth.

"The doctor tried to persuade me to go into the GP unit. He said it was 'homely' and I could do just what I wanted there. But there's a vast difference between someone else's place being 'homely' and my own home."

If you are considered sufficiently low risk to be allowed to give birth in any of these small maternity units, however, you might also think about the option of home birth. Birth centres, GP units and midwife clinics are for women who are expected to have normal births, and if it is a sensible choice to give birth in a unit like this, it is equally safe, or even safer, to give birth at home.

One of the strongest arguments against having your baby anywhere else is that once a woman is in an institution interventions can take place that no midwife or doctor would be likely to attempt at home. Even in small maternity units there is a risk that physiological labour is turned into managed labour just because you are in a place where medical hardware may be available, and where professionals make the decisions.

AT HOME

The essential difference between giving birth at home and giving birth in even the most peaceful, pleasant birth room in an institution is the knowledge that home is your space, the place that you control, and where other people come as guests.

"I went to my doctor expecting opposition and he said, 'What a good idea!'"

There is a genuine friendship with a doctor who shares your conviction that home is the best place, and who supports you.

If you have decided that you will feel more secure, more confident, and more relaxed giving birth at home, the first step is to find out what is available in your area. In Britain *you do not require a doctor's consent to have a home birth*. You can make arrangements directly with a midwife. But, unless you live in a place where there are keen home birth midwives, arranging a home birth may not be easy. You then have to ask yourself: Can I summon up the stamina, courage, and persistence to overcome obstacles that are likely to be put in my way? Where can I obtain the emotional support and practical help from other people that I shall need? Can I be assertive enough to state what I want, avoiding both aggression and submission, and to negotiate the care that I believe is right for me and my baby?

" 'You do realize', he said, 'that home birth is child abuse? We've got a perfectly good hospital here offering family-centred care.' "

The first challenge may be to obtain information about who can help if you meet refusal. One of the organizations listed on page 196 will be able to put you in touch with a group in your area. Working your way past other people's non-comprehension, their criticism, and their sometimes punitive responses, may be rather like finding your way through a baffling maze. But it can also be exciting!

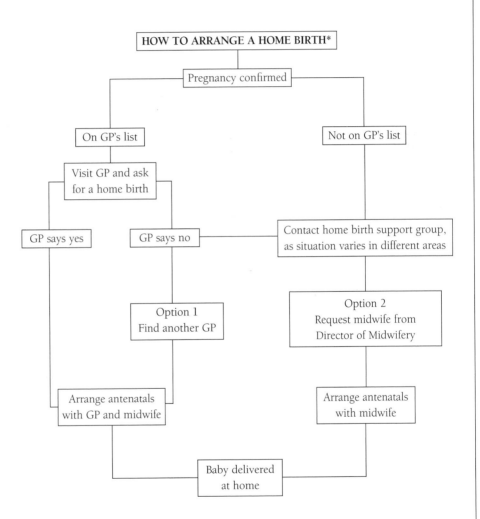

HOW TO ARRANGE A HOME BIRTH*

- Pregnancy confirmed
- On GP's list → Visit GP and ask for a home birth
- Not on GP's list
- GP says yes
- GP says no → Contact home birth support group, as situation varies in different areas
- Option 1 Find another GP
- Option 2 Request midwife from Director of Midwifery
- Arrange antenatals with GP and midwife
- Arrange antenatals with midwife
- Baby delivered at home

Being assertive
Do not attempt to broach the subject when you are flat on your back with your legs in the air. Make certain that you are sitting face to face with the doctor. Settle back comfortably in the chair, avoid fiddling nervously with your clothes, hands, or bag, and look the doctor straight in the eye.

"The doctor told me he wouldn't do a home birth because 'my place on the – Committee would be in jeopardy,' and said, 'If you have a home delivery, everyone'll want one!'"

It is often a good idea to rehearse what you are going to say beforehand with someone sympathetic. It helps to have someone who knows what doctors may say in these situations. Remember that most doctors are frightened of home births because they have no experience of them. You don't have to go into lengthy explanations or make a speech, to defend or excuse yourself, to quote statistics, or to placate the doctor. Refuse to be drawn into arguments. All you need do is say clearly and firmly that you want a home birth, and, if you wish, give a simple explanation of why. You may have to repeat it over and over again, a technique sometimes known as "the cracked record". Afterwards discuss with the other person how you each felt at different stages of the conversation, and at the end of it.

If you find this difficult, you can rehearse the interview by yourself, sitting in front of a mirror. Talk as if to the doctor, smiling and saying: "I should like a home birth." Then pause and listen attentively, imagining your doctor's reply. Then repeat your statement. Try this ten times. How did you sound . . . and look? Were you inclined to shout or whisper? Did you cross your arms so that you looked on the defensive? It is not only what you say, but how you say it, that is important. Your tone of voice can convey confidence or invite conflict or bullying. Practise saying, "I've decided that I want a home birth," in as many different ways as possible and settle for the tone and low pitch that makes you sound pleasantly assertive and friendly.

"None of the local GPs was prepared to take me on, and we were summoned to see the chief obstetrician of the area, who underlined that a home birth was out of the question. We politely said that we should have been grateful for expert assistance at the delivery but, since this was not forthcoming, we preferred to take our chances at home. Several weeks later, out of the blue, a letter arrived informing us that three midwives had been assigned to us."

Once you get approval in principle, most doctors will want to know that you will agree to be transferred to hospital if there are signs that the baby is over-stressed. You can make it clear that you agree to this, provided that everything is explained to you and you don't feel that any decisions are being taken over your head. You may want to say that there are obviously situations in which this would be your choice too, but that you would not want to transfer to hospital just because labour was long and drawn-out. Be sure to keep copies of all correspondence concerning your request for a home birth.

For a woman who is disabled, home may be the best place because it is familiar, and she can feel free in a setting that she knows well and which is adapted to her needs. A woman with polyarthritis says, "A lot of disabled women are told, 'You're disabled, so of course you go into hospital.' You don't get any choice at all. But I'm assertive – when you've been in a wheelchair for two years, you know how to get your own way." She was firm that she wanted a home birth and a birth pool, and found this the ideal solution. "Water encourages you to relax when you're disabled, and you're much freer in water. I just floated, with my boyfriend in the pool supporting me from behind. When we needed the midwives, they were

"What is important is the attitude you have to authority. To have a home birth, you have to be willing to question and to challenge authority."

there. When we wanted to be alone, we could be alone." She gave birth to a baby who rotated from the posterior position just before delivery, she had an intact perineum, and her baby was vigorously healthy and alert from the moment of birth.

If your doctor proposes a "compromise" solution – that you go into hospital for a short time and return home after a few hours, or are booked for a birth room, or suggests that care is modified to meet your special requests about not having drugs, or that electronic fetal monitoring will be used for only 20 minutes or so after you are admitted, and then you will be free to move around – and if you are not happy with that proposed compromise, say so and openly restate what you want.

"When you have a home birth, you don't have to go to someone else's place. It's your place. That makes all the difference."

On the other hand you may not want to say yes or no on the spot, and you can take time to think about it, discuss it with your partner, and then write to the doctor if you say, "I'd like a few days to consider that," "We need to talk this through," or "I'll think hard about that and let you know my decision next week." Do not be steam-rollered into an agreement that you may regret later.

Having said this, you do not have to put on a perfect performance. You have a right to be emotional, to get angry, to weep, to make mistakes, to be illogical, and even, if that is how it turns out, to be unassertive!

You are entitled to your own ideas about how you would like your birth to be. You are not on trial. You want the best for you and your baby. Whatever advice you are given, whatever the strength of other people's feelings, you have the right and responsibility to come to your own informed decision about where you have your baby.

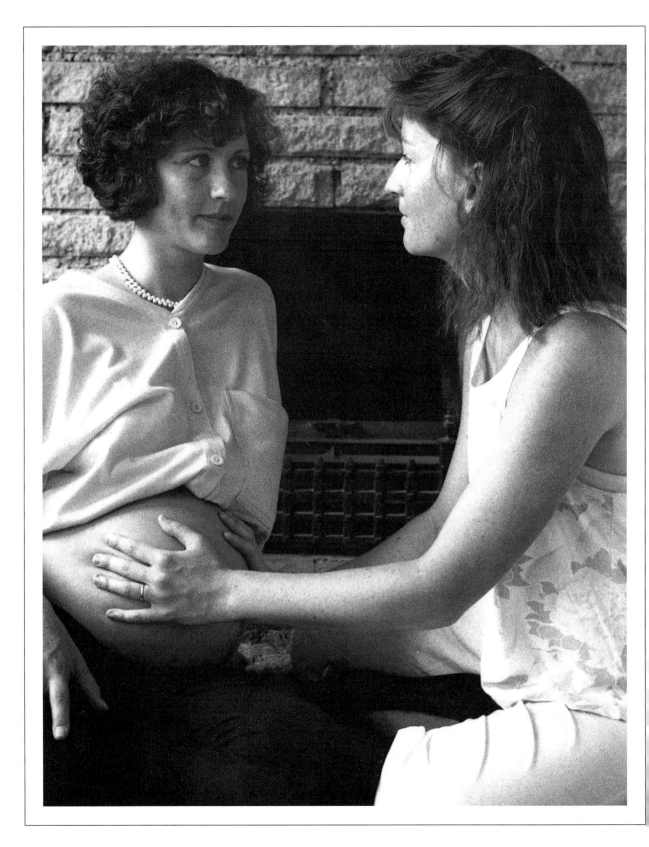

5

Your Midwife

A midwife is quite distinct from a nurse, though midwives have often trained as nurses before training as midwives. In some countries such as the Netherlands, Denmark and France, there is "direct entry" for most midwives. They do not have to be nurses first, but go straight into midwifery education. In others, such as Australia, they must be nurses first. Britain has a mix of nurse–midwives and direct entry midwives. Direct entry ensures that a midwife's main focus is on birth as a normal life event, rather than a disease and malfunction.

THE ROLE OF MIDWIVES

There is a handful of countries with no organized midwifery system at all: Panama, El Salvador, Venezuela, Colombia, Honduras, the Dominican Republic, and Burundi. Alone of all Western industrialized countries, Canada has been without a legal midwifery system of any kind until now, when midwifery is newly recognized and training is being developed in Ontario; there are also plans for midwife training to go ahead in Alberta and British Columbia.

Midwives are practitioners in their own right and are the only people whose training is concerned solely with caring for women in childbirth. Obstetricians are first and foremost gynaecologists, and their status comes from this rather than from baby-catching. Any doctor is legally allowed to deliver babies, even those with no special training. Indeed in a modern hospital many doctors with obstetric training have never had a chance to see a birth without intervention of any kind, since even in straightforward labours interventions such as artificial rupture of the membranes, withholding food and fluids from women, and the use of intravenous drips are standard practices. So some doctors see their involvement with childbirth as limited to dealing with abnormalities and complications.

In some countries, such as Britain, midwives have a statutory duty to attend a woman in childbirth when called, wherever the mother is. It is a woman's right to give birth where she chooses, and she does not need to book with a doctor for maternity care. Nor does she require a doctor's permission to give birth at home. She, or someone else on her behalf, must summon midwife help, however, once labour is underway, or as soon as possible after the birth.

Traditional midwifery

Midwives have a long history of persecution going back to the Middle Ages, when many were burned as witches. In North America the midwives who arrived with the waves of migration in the 19th century came to be dismissed as relics of an outmoded life-style and of European traditions in childbirth, on which migrants had turned their backs in favour of modern medicine. Where in the early years of the 20th century most women were cared for in their own homes by midwives and family doctors, by the 1940s this had changed to hospital care by doctors, with nurses doing the minor tasks. In remote areas, where few doctors wanted to work, midwifery continued to be practised. The 1970s saw a rebirth of midwifery in North America, against strong medical opposition.

For a midwife to attend birth is in many cases against the law. It is a radical act. There is an underground midwifery, and midwives constantly risk imprisonment for practising medicine without a licence and, if a baby dies, for manslaughter or even murder. While some states now register or license midwives, in others the practice of midwifery is still regarded as a crime.

Doctors in North America oppose midwifery because they believe it is dangerous and it threatens their profession and their incomes. Many obstetricians are of the opinion that midwifery offers mothers sub-standard care: "Why settle for a Ford when you can have a Cadillac?" They see themselves as the Cadillacs of birth. It is only in North America, and in hospitals elsewhere that are based on the American model, that obstetric nurses are used in place of midwives, and that the word "midwife" suggests outdated care by old grannies.

Actually some of those granny midwives were very good. There is much that we can learn from the traditional practice of midwifery in rural areas, not only in North America, but anywhere in the world where women healers are part of a long tradition of helping women through the biological transitions of their lives, and in assisting not only at each person's coming to birth, but also at the surrendering of life.

Midwifery today

The modern, professionally trained midwife is a specialist in childbearing, qualified to take responsibility for women antenatally, through the birth itself, and for four weeks afterwards. She has specific skills to support the physiological process, to understand deviations from the normal, and to know when obstetric advice or assistance is required. Unlike the obstetrician, the main focus of her interest is the normal, not the pathological, and the whole woman rather than one organ, the uterus. Midwives working outside hospital resort to intervention less readily than hospital midwives, because events that would be considered abnormal according to the paradigm of standard hospital labour are considered normal away from the rigid protocols of the hospital.

Hospital midwives have tended to become subordinate members of teams headed by obstetricians, and have been powerless to prevent this. They are used to control people waiting in the antenatal clinic, to do menial jobs such as weighing women and putting a stick in a urine sample to note whether it changes colour, to chaperone doctors when they do a vaginal examination, to prepare equipment for the obstetrician to perform an intervention in labour and to clean up afterwards, to keep records, and in

"The great advantage of home birth is that the labour is undisturbed. The woman does not have to be moved, and the surroundings are familiar. I don't have all the paperwork that I must do in hospital, and we are all more relaxed."
A midwife

some countries where there are too many doctors – such as Italy – to be the doctor's assistant at the birth. Sweden and the Netherlands, both countries with very few baby deaths, are notable exceptions to this trend, and in each midwives have retained their professional integrity, with nearly all of the Swedish midwives working in hospitals, but most Dutch midwives doing home births.

Some midwives quite like being absorbed into hospital systems and do not want more responsibility. Others feel that the freedom to exercise their skills has been eroded. In hospitals women are often seen by junior doctors – house officers or "interns" – who are learning about obstetrics, and who make decisions about care which might be very different from those made by an experienced midwife standing by. Indeed she may also feel that many interventionist procedures are being carried out unnecessarily by some of the senior doctors and obstetricians.

So midwives are in a difficult position. Some opt for security in a hospital system and do not step out of line. Others fight that system from the inside. Still others decide to serve women outside hospital and attend home births and work in birth centres although, to do this, they may have to become independent, private midwives – in most countries separate from the standard health service. In the Netherlands independent midwifery is the norm, and midwives are on a professional par with general practitioners. About 70 per cent of them work outside hospitals and 16 per cent in hospitals. (The rest are in clinics, midwifery schools, research, and so on.) In Italy, in contrast, the vast majority work in hospitals and only a handful are independent. For most Italian women, except those in cities such as Florence, Rome, Genoa, and Turin, who are seeking home birth in increasing numbers, it is a sign of poverty to go to a midwife.*

You can find out about independent midwives from the organizations listed on page 196.

THE MIDWIFE AND HOME BIRTH

For a midwife who has worked only in hospitals, it can be threatening to take on a home birth. The worst mistake she can make is to try to move the hospital to the home and attempt to practise exactly as she would in hospital. She needs to think through how she is going to support the woman so that there is the greatest chance of labour progressing naturally at its own pace and in its own way.

"As a midwife I would never persuade a woman to have a home birth. She's got to be very sure that it's what she wants. But I am certain that the majority of complications arise purely because women are in hospital."

"I have learned most about birth from midwives."
A doctor

A midwife's responsibilities

Anxiety is contaminating. Anyone who is apprehensive around a woman in labour communicates his or her own fear, and can have a negative effect on the labour. It is the responsibility of the midwife to face up to and explore her fears well in advance of attending a home birth, and to share them with colleagues who are experienced and working outside hospital, so that she does not bring infectious anxiety with her to a birth. It helps if she has already attended births outside hospital as an assistant to an experienced midwife. This is the most practical way of learning the art.

When a midwife attends in quiet confidence, she is able to tolerate inaction and can watch and wait on this child's coming to life, giving the mother of her own strength and inner joy. She blends with the surroundings, merging with the pattern of that woman's life. She does not take charge or take over. She does not "manage" labour: in many ways her task is a more difficult one than this. It demands great strength of personality. She needs to observe minutely and with sensitive awareness everything that is happening in the labour and to be aware of what is happening in the mind of the woman she is attending.

A baby may weigh three kilos or five kilos and still be of normal birth weight. In the same way a labour can be completely normal and yet be far from average. Dilatation may be slow or very rapid. The woman may have an overwhelming desire to push or almost none at all. Expulsion may take ten minutes or four hours. There may be lulls and rest phases. Each labour has its rhythm, its own cadences, which make it different from all others.

A good midwife understands when she should stand back and let things unfold, and knows when she needs to intervene. And the interventions are rare. Far more often she gives quiet, tender support to the woman in her care, simply allowing the energy of birth to sweep through the mother's body, and helping her to find strength within herself. When you stand watching a river in full flood, you know that you cannot fight its power. But you can use it so that its flow sweeps you onwards.

A woman should be able to expect open and honest communication with the midwife. Instead of "reassurance" there is frank explanation, exploring of options, a genuine sharing between the two women, which goes far beyond the trite phrases that are sometimes trotted out in an attempt to keep a patient docile and placid.

When a woman and her midwife relate to each other with mutual respect, warmth, and openness, it is as if they are on a journey together in which exciting discoveries are made, their understanding deepens, and they are both enriched by the birth experience.

"All midwives are based at our hospital . . . When I started labour, my husband had to go and fetch the midwives from the hospital (I suppose they were without cars). On his arrival the Night Sister greeted him with 'Couldn't you persuade her to come in? It would be much safer' . . . It was good to be at home but, if there can be such a thing, it was a hospitalized home confinement. They turned our bedroom into a hospital. Everything was timed, recorded, methodical, sterile."

A good midwife loves women. She does not dominate, direct, or even instruct. The word "midwife" is Anglo-Saxon for "with woman". The midwife is side by side and with the woman. Except on the rare occasions when she needs to take decisive action to avert danger, she follows rather than leads. Ina May Gaskin, spiritual midwife at The Farm, the alternative-style community in Tennessee, says, "Pregnant and birthing mothers are elemental forces, in the same way that gravity, thunderstorms, earthquakes, and hurricanes are elemental forces. In order to understand the laws of their energy flow, you have to love and respect them for their magnificence, at the same time that you study them with the accuracy of a true scientist."*

When women give birth in hospital, they often apologize to their midwives. Mavis Kirkham, a midwife researcher, wrote of a hospital research project, "Most of the women I observed in labour apologized. Many apologized frequently if they felt they were not behaving well or were 'being a nuisance', or 'causing trouble' by making requests or simply receiving routine care from busy staff. The commonest words I heard women say immediately after delivery were 'I'm sorry . . .' "* When women placate authority in this way, their deference is implicit acknowledgement of an institutional power structure in which they are at the lowest level. They are, in effect, intruders on the professional territory of the hospital. If midwives accept these apologies, they too acknowledge and submit to this power structure. A good midwife does not criticize or judge the woman in her care, and even though a woman may be submissive and seek approval, she helps her to stand on her own feet and to find the locus of control that is *inside herself*.

A good midwife is not only someone who delivers a baby. She is midwife to a woman's transformation to motherhood and a man's transformation to fatherhood. She is midwife to all the dreams and hopes surrounding the coming to being of that child, and to the process of maturing and growth that is involved for both parents.

Meeting your midwife
Even though midwifery is the foundation of care in childbirth throughout Europe, and the whole system would collapse if midwives walked out, most countries no longer provide any continuity in care. Different groups of midwives work in the antenatal clinic, the labour and delivery rooms, and on the postpartum ward. At a time in their lives when women are at their most vulnerable, they meet total strangers. In Britain attempts are being made – through the creation of midwife teams who get to know the mothers in their care during pregnancy – to deal with this problem of

You are the midwife of my hopes *by Keith Eisner*
The male partner of a midwife wrote this poem about the woman he loves:

You are the midwife of my hopes.
I'm not just talking about the safe world contained
in the snapshot
Of the new baby on the new blanket
(or the cleanly typed story ready to mail)
Or the picture of you and the parents
looking tired,
looking triumphant

But the times
when no one's taking pictures,
when you're alone beyond
the light of the lamps
in someone else's bedroom
the guide in someone else's
dream.
And, alternately, you taste
the sweetness of their faith
and the sour mash of their fear.

"Take me to the hospital,"
says the mother.
"I want drugs," she says.
She looks out of her pain
and into you and says,
as I have said,
(so many times)
"I'm not strong enough."
"I can't do this."
Everyone says,
"Yes, you can, you're doing fine,"
but there are few poets as good as you
who can make language enter the blood
and touch the heart.

I don't know how you do it.
You say the same words others say

But your words carry the conviction
of having passed

through muscle and bone,
success and failure:
"You are strong" you say,
"You are strong."
"It won't be long," you tell her
and she believes you even though
she's in that place
where there's no day and no night.
She holds your hand
as another contraction begins
and looks into your eyes:
"It won't be long."

It doesn't always work –
Sometimes the woman goes to the hospital.
Sometimes I choose to fail.
Sometimes you walk through the hospital parking lot
with your head down,
softly pounding your fists on your thighs.
Or we sleep with a space
between our backs;
the bones of sweet words
crumbled in our mouths.

But most of the time it does work.
You know how to wait.
You know the hard, unyielding
business of giving birth
and having hope.

You can't push for the mothers
or for me.
We do it ourselves.
But you are there
hours for her,
years for me.
You drop down beneath our skins
to love and wait

You are the midwife of my hopes.

A MIDWIFE'S VISIT

For any woman who only meets her midwife when she is admitted to hospital in labour, and who then may find that this person disappears with the next shift change, the experience of bearing a child is bound to be fragmented and depersonalized. When a woman gets to know her midwife during pregnancy and the two become friends, a bond of understanding develops, and the emotional support the midwife gives can help the mother feel confident and strong.

The midwife hears the baby's heart through a Pinard's stethoscope.

She traces the baby's body with her hands and talks to the mother about what they can both feel.

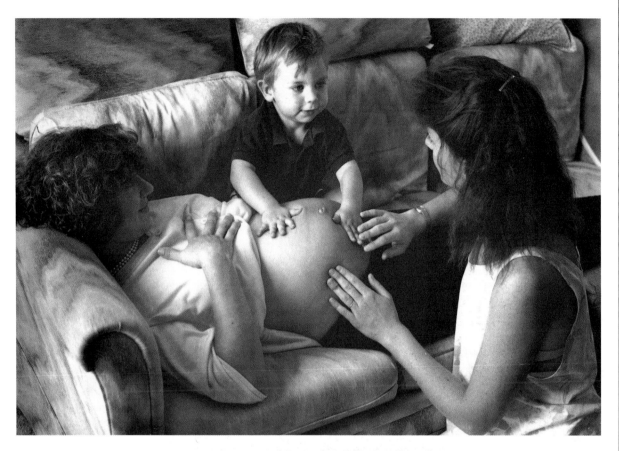

It is fun for the older child too. He learns about how babies are born in the most natural way possible, is shown how to feel the firm curve of the baby's bottom, and is delighted when a little foot kicks against his hand. The new baby will not come as a surprise or as an alien invader, but is someone whom he has already learned about and even touched.

The midwife fixes the blood pressure cuff and starts to blow it up. The child is intrigued as she explains it, and then enjoys having a go himself. This kind of relationship with a child is much easier when antenatal care takes place at home, so that the older child is in a familiar environment and on his own ground, and the midwife comes as a friend of the family.

anonymity, which is frustrating and often confusing for midwives as well as mothers. But only in Denmark and the Netherlands is it the norm to have continuity of care from your own midwife. In southern Europe doctors have totally taken over antenatal care, and even in countries where midwife care at birth is the normal system, a woman who is having her baby in hospital may never meet the midwives assigned to her until she is admitted in labour. Having your baby outside hospital may be your only opportunity to get to know your midwife.

Questions to ask

At your first meetings with the midwife, or with the small group of midwives who are attending you, there will be many questions to ask. If you are choosing an independent midwife, you will need to put these questions before you can come to a firm arrangement with each other. Either way, you won't want to fire questions at her, but can incorporate many of these into your discussion with her. Here are some of the questions that you may like to bear in mind:

☐ How long has she been a midwife?

☐ Why did she become a midwife?

☐ What was her training?

☐ How many mothers has she delivered, and of these how many were home births or not in a large hospital?

☐ Does she work alone or with other midwives?

☐ If she works alone, what happens if two women she has booked are in labour at the same time?

☐ If she works with other midwives, will you be able to meet them?

☐ What is her back-up system? Does she work closely with any doctors?

☐ What does she carry with her in terms of equipment and supplies? Does she carry any drugs, for example, for pain relief and to stimulate the uterus?

☐ What resuscitation equipment for the baby does she carry?

☐ What antenatal care does she provide? Are there any home visits?

☐ Does she offer childbirth classes or pregnancy discussion groups? If not, what classes does she recommend?

☐ What postnatal care does she provide?

☐ What does she do if a woman has a very long labour?

☐ What is the plan of action if transfer to hospital should be necessary?

☐ Under what conditions does she transfer; what are her transfer rates?

☐ If she works in a birth centre or GP unit, are there any standard procedures that must be followed regarding admission and when you are in labour, such as compulsory fetal monitoring, birth positions, and so on?

☐ What are her views on routine episiotomy? What is her episiotomy rate?

☐ How often do her mothers have an intact perineum?

☐ What happens if your perineum requires suturing? Will she do this herself or call a doctor?

☐ When are her holidays? If she plans to go on holiday towards the end of your pregnancy or within three weeks after you are due, and you go into labour, whom should you call?

Other things you may wish to talk with her about are: nutrition in pregnancy, the people you would like to have with you at the birth, your thoughts about fetal monitoring, moving around in labour, birth positions, exactly what help she gives a mother in order to avoid the need for episiotomy, her basic beliefs about birth, and breastfeeding. Discuss with her exactly what you are hoping for with this birth.

If you are booking an independent midwife, you will also want to ask her fee, when it should be paid, and what is included.

After you have met, one of the most important questions of all for *you* to answer is whether you like her as a person and feel relaxed and confident with her. Can you be completely open about how you feel and what you want? Talk with other women for whom she has cared to find out about their experience with her. You can learn a great deal from them.

"She was wonderful . . . She visited me at home in the early stages of my pregnancy, and chatted as a friend would over a cup of coffee . . . As my pregnancy progressed, she called at the house once a week for her own personal check-up. She made friends with my three-year-old, letting her feel my tummy and listen to the baby's heartbeat."

Any woman who chooses to become a midwife cares deeply for other women and loves babies. Yet midwives working in hospitals have often learned to guard their feelings and have been forced to hold back from giving themselves completely. They have been warned not to "become emotionally involved with the patient". When a midwife works in a different environment, outside the rigid hospital system, she is free to be herself and to have a close, caring relationship with a woman whom she comes to know, not as a patient, but as a sister.

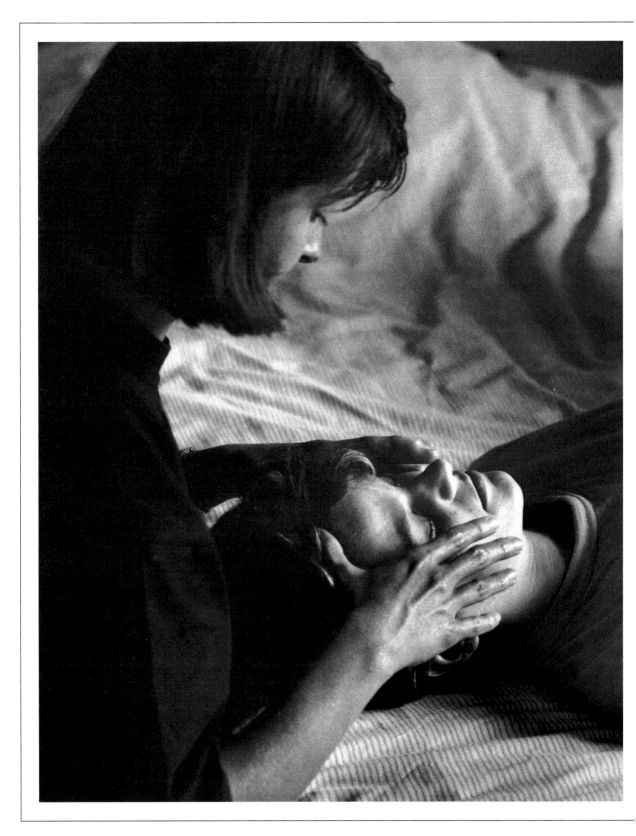

6

Getting Ready

Now that you have made the decision to give birth out of hospital, there are preparations you can make for it to be the best experience possible. The chances of a safe, happy birth are enormously increased if you approach labour healthy, energetic, well-nourished, and self-confident, and if you understand how to help yourself by learning movements that allow your body to open up, and know how to relax and breathe rhythmically.

YOUR ANTENATAL CARE

The fragmentation of care that often occurs in hospital clinics results from different staff members performing different tests as women are shuffled from one line of chairs to another, from room to room, from cubicle to cubicle, from person to person.

Yet, even if you escape being screened by a variety of anonymous doctors, nurses, midwives, and radiographers, you are still not receiving good antenatal care if you have tests that detract from, or take the place of, your caregivers' relationship with you as a unique, individual human being. Antenatal care should be far more than screening for abnormalities. You need holistic care. I mean by this that you are cared for as a whole person, rather than merely tested for potential problems.

Even if a woman has only one professional caregiver, or a small group of caregivers, the medical model rather than the holistic model of care is often adopted. It entails turning her into a patient and dividing up information about her body so that it can be laid out on a record card: blood pressure, weight, urine, haemoglobin, and height of fundus. Her hopes, her fears, the stresses of her daily life, financial worries, conflicts in the family, problems at work – these social and emotional aspects of pregnancy are seen as irrelevant compared with physical symptoms that can be checked, enumerated, and recorded.

Many investigations that are unnecessary take place in antenatal clinics today. Some are potentially harmful. Since the early years of the century, when modern obstetric-style antenatal care was first introduced, tests have proliferated. Doctors seem to be under the impression that any item of information might come in useful sometime, somehow. But information is useless unless it affects the kind of care that is provided.

Midwives in many traditional cultures were giving antenatal care long before the 20th century, visiting the pregnant woman's home to teach her about pregnancy, to discuss diet, work, and exercise, to massage her with oil and palpate her uterus, to talk with her about her husband and family, to ward off danger with shared religious rites and prayers, and to make plans for the birth. Traditional midwives have usually been far more than birth attendants. They control the mysterious passage between the world of shadows and ancestors and the world of life. Throughout Europe, Asia, and South America they have usually had an important role in helping the pregnant woman to create balance and harmony in her mind and body. It is often expressed as yin and yang, or in terms of the concepts of heat and cold, as in the medieval theory of humours.

"I have to go on the bus to get to the clinic, as I haven't a car. The journey takes 45 minutes each way, and I usually have to wait at least half an hour. I have two – perhaps three – minutes with the doctor. The only reason I go is because I'd worry that something was going wrong if I didn't."

"The midwife came to see me at home and spent a lot of time talking about what I wanted. She became a friend and we all look forward to her visits."

"He said, 'The baby's very small, you know. Try and eat more.' Next time I saw another doctor, who told me, 'You've got a good-sized baby there. It's going to be a whopper!' I don't know what to believe. Should I be stuffing myself to try and make the baby bigger or will it be so huge that it can't get out?"

Today obstetricians construct the agenda for antenatal care. As we have seen already, there is strong evidence that other influences on pregnant women – the socio-economic conditions that result in inequalities in health – usually have more effect on the outcome of pregnancy than anything that the most dedicated of obstetricians can do in an antenatal clinic. Socially deprived women, who are most in need of care, are the ones who are most likely to delay seeking it. A woman with a ten-month-old baby and a two-and-a-half-year-old child, no help at home, nobody else to care for the children, and no private transport, may find it difficult to attend an antenatal clinic even though it is only two or three miles away. A teenager who is hoping against hope that she is not pregnant, trying to hide it from her family, and with no idea of how to get help, is unlikely to find her way to the antenatal clinic until pregnancy is well-advanced.

It is much safer to have a baby if you are educated and well-off than if you are uneducated and poor. In England and Wales perinatal mortality rates are worked out on the basis of the husband's occupation. Twice as many babies die in social class 5, at the bottom of the scale, as in social class 1, at the top of it.*

Standard antenatal care entails up to 15 visits to a clinic or hospital, or a mixture of both, and a woman may encounter 50 or more different professionals, many of whom are bound to make conflicting comments and give contradictory advice. Far from providing reassurance, these encounters serve only to increase anxiety.

Routine antenatal tests

There is no point in having tests unless their results are going to affect care. Useless information provided by routine tests is often employed as a charm against a perilous passage, in the same way that talismans have been used traditionally by pregnant women to guard against evil. With modern antenatal care this information is often not even conveyed to the mother, but is retained by the doctor and recorded, as part of a series of illegible hieroglyphs resembling mystic runes, in case-notes that are sometimes not even passed on to the other caregivers.

"It was a shambles really. The doctor gave me the wrong card. It was a different blood group, and it said 'Rhesus negative' but I am Rhesus positive. I didn't realize till much later, but I could have had a whole lot of treatment I didn't need, and the other woman, who had my card, wouldn't have had treatment that she needed. At least they let us keep our own records. If the clinic had kept them, it might never have been found out."

The results of most tests have a margin of error that is often very wide and can lead to false negative and false positive diagnoses. False *negative* diagnosis suggests that there is no problem when in fact there is one. False *positive* diagnosis appears to reveal a problem when there is none. Both are dangerous. The first gives rise to complacency in the face of special risk. The second causes needless anxiety, and may lead to unnecessary interventions, such as induction of labour or Caesarean section.

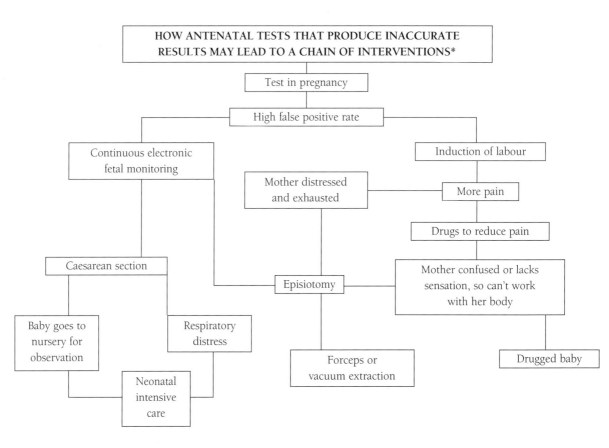

HOW ANTENATAL TESTS THAT PRODUCE INACCURATE RESULTS MAY LEAD TO A CHAIN OF INTERVENTIONS*

☐ There is nothing to be gained from regularly testing urine for sugar in pregnancy unless you are diabetic. A trace of sugar in urine is very common. It may simply mean that you have recently eaten something especially sweet. Bananas sometimes have this effect.

☐ Routine weighing is a waste of time too. Weight checks give useful information only if you started pregnancy very underweight or very overweight. The baby's growth is better assessed by having one or two caregivers regularly palpate your uterus so that they are in touch, literally, with the baby's development and are in a position to know whether this development is consistent with *your* pregnancy as a whole.

☐ Vaginal examinations are usually unnecessary. In some countries, including the USA, they are performed weekly starting at 37 weeks. In Britain one vaginal examination is often done routinely some time between 33 and 37 weeks. However, vaginal examinations increase the risk of infection and premature rupture of the membranes and, because of this, Caesarean section.*

☐ Ultrasound enables obstetricians to visualize the baby in the uterus and learn much more about fetal development, and it reveals certain abnormalities. If you have a scan at around 16 weeks, the date of conception, and hence the expected date of delivery, can be estimated fairly accurately, *but* only within two weeks. If you are unsure about the date you conceived, you might decide that this is a good reason for choosing to have a scan. On the other hand, the baby will be born when it is ready. If you have already had a low-birth-weight baby, you may also want to monitor fetal growth with several ultrasound scans. But diagnosis of the baby's weight based on fundal height is almost as accurate as that from ultrasound, so whether or not you have a series of scans is up to you.*

☐ Biochemical tests of fetal wellbeing proliferated in the 70s and 80s. They included alpha-feta-protein testing, measurement of HCG (human chorionic gonadotrophin), placental proteins, HPL (human placental lactogen) and oestrogen levels with 24-hour urine specimens, blood tests, or, occasionally, measurement of levels in the saliva. A small proportion of the biochemical tests available can be useful in early pregnancy to screen for abnormalities. But all the tests that are employed later in pregnancy to try to predict low birth weight, premature birth, or stillbirth are a waste of time.*

☐ Cardiotocography – fetal heart-rate monitoring in pregnancy – has certainly added to obstetricians' knowledge about life inside the uterus, but four randomized controlled trials have not demonstrated any direct benefit for mothers and babies themselves. So you may decide that it is not worth having this test.*

Holistic antenatal care

If you are having holistic antenatal care, you will be offered only those screening procedures that are likely to give useful information and make a difference in the care that is given during pregnancy or at the birth. While being alert to the possibility of pathology, its main focus is woman-centred.

A holistic approach enables you to care for yourself, instead of just being at the receiving end of care. It is concerned with feelings and relationships that are important to you rather than merely with physiology. And it helps you to grow in self-awareness, in self-confidence, and in strength. Holistic antenatal care is empowering.

For care to be holistic, it is essential to have a continuing relationship with a few caregivers only, who get to know you well and who make time at each visit to obtain full and accurate information, and to talk freely, in a totally accepting atmosphere. There is genuine sharing.

NUTRITION

Everything you eat during pregnancy should enhance your feeling of wellbeing and be good for you and the baby. Choose wholegrain bread and cereals, fruit and vegetables – freshly picked whenever you can get them – and to ensure a good supply of vitamin C have one raw fruit or vegetable meal every day. Eat some protein at each meal, either in the form of meat, fish, dairy products (such as cheese, milk, and yogurt), a soya bean product such as tofu, or a mix of pulses (peas, beans, or lentils) and grains (bread, rice, or pasta). Ensure that you have ample supplies of iron by eating iron-rich foods: leafy green vegetables and egg yolks are good sources. Use olive oil, sunflower oil and other polyunsaturated oils as a large proportion of your fats, and enjoy the sugar in fresh and dried fruit, rather than adding sugar to desserts.

An excess of any one type of food is bound to be bad for you. It is possible, for example, to have carrot poisoning, and even to die of it. And plenty of people have had coronaries associated with eating, among other things, excessive quantities of meat and dairy foods.

When considering your diet in pregnancy, think about the foods you enjoy most. It may be a good idea to write them down. Then look at what you have written to see if any of them do not measure up to your standards of nutrition. Are there any junk foods? Do they contain artificial colourings or are they full of preservatives? Do any provide empty calories? Are there too many fatty foods? There are fun foods like popcorn and crisps, and foods that make you feel indulged and cosseted like whipped-cream cakes or a box of Belgian chocolates, instant foods like a Chinese take-away or pot noodles, foods that warm you up on a bitterly cold day – cake, doughnuts, and hot puddings, for example – and other foods, like ice cream, that make you feel cool in the heat. If you are particularly fond of food which you know is not good for you, you might then list what you especially like about it: salty, crunchy, crisp, sweet, smooth, filling, quick to make, cheap, reminds me of home (or Rome, or Vienna, or somewhere else). Invariably, there are alternatives that bring a similar sense of wellbeing.

When you look at what you enjoy about the foods that are not so good for you, think how you can find the same qualities in more nutritious foods. If you want an instant food, choose a bowl of nuts and raisins, bite into a banana or apple, or bake a potato in the microwave. If you long for something hot and satisfying, a pan of home-made soup heated up on the stove is much more nutritious, and probably tastier and more satisfying, than a mug of hot chocolate.

At the end of pregnancy many women become constipated, and this can be treated by increasing your carbohydrate intake – eating more wholegrain bread and muesli, for example. But this is effective only if you also cut your fat intake to the minimum.

Despite the advice often given to omit salt in order to prevent pre-eclampsia, there is no convincing evidence that salt restriction is effective in achieving this. A study of 2,000 pregnant women, half of whom were recommended to increase salt, and the other half to avoid it, revealed that there were significantly fewer women with pre-eclampsia in the high-salt group.* Nor do you need to force yourself to eat large quantities of high-protein foods, since an excessive amount of protein can reduce a baby's birth weight.*

In an overview of all the studies of nutrition in pregnancy, the head of the epidemiology programme at the Human Nutrition Research Center on Ageing at Tuft's University in Massachusetts concludes: "There can be no rational justification for either allowing pregnant women to go hungry or for imposing either dietary restrictions or marked manipulation of the dietary constituents upon them."*

MEDICATION

You will know already that it is wise to avoid drugs in pregnancy unless you really need them. But there can be few hard and fast rules, and it is usually a question of weighing up the risks and benefits of the drug against the risks and benefits of not treating a disease. Sometimes a pregnant woman has an illness that holds possible dangers for the baby. Then treating the illness is a sensible choice, even though it entails taking a drug. A high fever, for example, can cause miscarriage and, if the fever can't be brought down in any other way, it is probably better to take aspirin or paracetamol.

All dietary supplements, including vitamins and minerals, are drugs and may overload the system with one mineral or vitamin and thus result in nutritional deficiency. Some supplements – such as vitamins A and D – are toxic in high doses. So avoid mega-vitamins and, unless you know that you suffer from nutritional deficiencies that cannot be rectified by a change of diet, do not take supplementary vitamins and minerals.

A drug is not necessarily safe for pregnancy because it occurs naturally in the wild. Herbs are powerful, and they too can be poisonous. Most herbs prescribed by reputable herbalists – select one who is a member of an association of registered practitioners of alternative or complementary medicine – are safe, and may be a great help to you in keeping healthy and coping with discomforts in pregnancy. But there are others that may be teratogenic (causing congenital malformation), or that lead to miscarriage. Judy Priest, in her book *Drugs in Pregnancy**, lists the following herbs as potentially dangerous for anyone, whether pregnant or not: comfrey, berberis, ragwort, prickly ash, excessive intake of ginseng, feverfew, and the kernels of apricots, plums, and peaches.

Some herbs increase uterine muscle tone, so can be helpful in producing effective contractions in labour. But the same herbs used in pregnancy, in high doses and by women who are particularly vulnerable, may be associated with miscarriage. So it is wise to avoid herbs such as feverfew and pennyroyal.*

If you are healthy, you are unlikely to need iron supplements. An increased blood supply in pregnancy results in dilution of haemoglobin, and this often causes a quite normal drop in haemoglobin levels in blood of up to two grams per decilitre. This is a natural process that helps the flow of blood across the placenta to the baby. If your haemoglobin level does not fall beneath 11 grams per decilitre, there is no need for iron supplements.* Unnecessary iron supplementation can cause constipation that results in piles, and may result in macrocytosis, where red blood cells enlarge and become sticky so that they cannot flow through fine capillaries, impairing circulation.

In the late 70s it was discovered that very high haemoglobin levels in pregnancy are associated with low birth weight. So there is a disadvantage in artificially boosting your haemoglobin level unless it is known that you are definitely anaemic.*

It is in the interest of pharmaceutical companies who manufacture vitamin and mineral supplements to sell them as widely as possible and to persuade doctors that their patients need them. There is no reason why any pregnant woman should be dosed with these simply as a matter of routine, however, and vitamins and minerals are best obtained from a well-balanced diet with plenty of fresh fruit and vegetables, wholegrain cereals, and protein in the form of milk and milk products, pulses, and – for non-vegetarians – small quantities of meat and fish.

EXERCISE

Regular exercise that you really enjoy helps you feel positive about your pregnant body, tones your muscles, and whips up the circulation. Swimming is excellent, because it is so easy to move when floating in water that takes your weight. Brisk walking in the countryside or a park is good

You can devise your own exercise and relaxation routines. Many public pools offer women-only sessions.

too. Many women go to aerobic classes, but these should always be adapted to pregnancy. If any movement proves a strain or causes pain, drop it from the routine, and concentrate on easy, flowing, rhythmic movements instead.

Competitive games, in which you are inclined to ignore the messages of tiredness and pain coming from your body because you are out to beat the other person, are not a good idea in pregnancy.

There is one form of dancing that is especially suitable: belly dancing – the slow, sinuous kind, rather than rapid gyrations with a diamond in your navel! Belly dancing was taught traditionally in North Africa as part of fertility rituals to mark a girl's passage to womanhood, and women attending a birth danced while the mother rolled her pelvis in a similar way during contractions. Any movement like this that frees the pelvis can help the baby's head to rotate and descend deep into the pelvis.

There is an exception to this. If your pelvic ligaments stretch too much in late pregnancy, so that you feel like a disjointed doll, have backache, and stumble often, pronounced pelvic movements that entail hollowing your lower back may make things worse. You should select only those movements that involve tightening your buttocks and abdominal muscles, gently releasing, and then tightening them again.

Special yoga classes for pregnancy are helpful too, since they include opening movements for the pelvis and, at the same time, help you find a focus of concentration inside yourself in a very satisfying way. The result is confidence and inner poise.

Many active birth classes are based on yoga. In these you learn movements to enable muscles to "give" and help your pelvis widen to let the baby through, practise a range of upright positions and movements, and discover how you can use your partner to support you in different positions during labour. Like yoga, these exercises also lead to improved physical coordination, increased self-confidence, and a sense of inner balance.

One of the best things about exercise is the healthy glow and sense of luxurious relaxation that comes *afterwards*. Give yourself time to enjoy that.

REST AND RELAXATION

You will get the most out of your pregnancy if you can take time to rest and nurture yourself. That means making a space in your life to do anything you like – to listen to music, to read, to dream, or to do nothing at all – a space free from the stress of striving to reach a goal, to live up to a standard, or to please someone else.

It is very difficult to do this when you have other children and little or no help with them, difficult to do if your partner dismisses domestic work as trivial and something he was never much good at anyway, and difficult if your job is the kind which consumes all your energy. Your own feelings of responsibility, and the guilt you feel when you are not meeting other people's expectations of you, may hold you back from creating this small, private citadel of time and space that is yours alone. But if you *can* do it, you will feel more "centred" and you will also be better able to relax and enjoy being pregnant.

I remember reading a short story in which the heroine was in labour: " 'I *must*. I *MUST* relax!' she muttered fiercely." The feeling that relaxation is compulsory, that if you don't manage to relax something awful will happen, and that you have to fight to achieve it, is not conducive to relaxation, and makes you more tense. Relaxation is a *luxury*.

If you are having your baby at home or in another out-of-hospital setting, relaxation is the basis of your preparation for birth. It is also a major protection against stress in pregnancy, and is invaluable after the baby comes, when you need to relax in order to breastfeed, as well as to make all the adjustments – the amazing leap across the great divide – entailed in becoming a parent.

It helps to have a quiet, peaceful place where you are least likely to be interrupted, and where, like an animal in her lair, you can go to ground. It might be your bed, the bath, a garden, a couch in front of an open fire, at the seashore or in a meadow. Any comfortable space where, if only for ten minutes, you will not be disturbed by the phone ringing or people demanding your attention, will do well.

First make a nest for yourself with cushions, perhaps a duvet, a beanbag, or some rolled-up towels or rugs. If you are in the bath, slip a small rolled towel behind your neck or use a Chinese neck cushion. If you are in a chair, on the ground, or in bed, either recline, well-supported with cushions, or lie down on your side.

In late pregnancy avoid lying flat on your back. Your heavy uterus tends to press on the *vena cava*, the large vein in the lower part of your body, in this position. This slows down the blood flow back to your heart and may make you feel sick and giddy, as well as restricting blood flow to the placenta, and oxygen to the baby. So, either sitting well-propped-up or lying on your side, support your head and neck with cushions and get comfortable. If you are on your side, a cushion under your upper knee often helps. If sitting up, you will need one in the small of your back. The first few times you do this, it is useful to have someone read the following passage for you, slowly, in a low-pitched voice.

> *Bend your arms and knees and let your body spread, taking as much space as possible. Release tension on a long breath out. Then let the breath flow in when you are ready for it. Don't suck air in. Just allow your lungs to fill. There is a slight pause, as when the crest of a wave is reached, after which you give another breath out, relaxing all down your back and right down to your toes as you do so.*
>
> *As you listen to the sound of your breathing, be aware of your whole body: your skin where it touches the air and the fabric of your clothing, the strong muscles underneath, your swelling uterus with the baby moving inside it, and the blood pulsing through your body.*
>
> *Are there any parts of your body that are holding on to tension? You may want to find a more comfortable position. Roll your head slightly forwards and round your shoulders. If you are not completely comfortable, have a stretch and re-settle. Or roll into a ball like a hedgehog, and then slowly uncurl until you feel at ease.*
>
> *As you continue, listen to your slow breathing and relax a little more with each breath out. Enjoy your breathing as if you were listening to waves on the seashore. Focus on the breath out, and you will find that the breath in looks after itself.*

To derive most advantage from relaxation, you need to practise it daily, setting aside a regular time for this self-nurturing. If you have the opportunity, take a rest after lunch, or perhaps in the evening when you return from work. But, even if you can do it only when you wake in the morning or go to bed at night, or if you wake to empty your bladder and find it difficult to get back to sleep, ten minutes' relaxation can give you the nurturing you need.

BREATHING

You will know how to breathe when you are in labour, just as you know how to breathe now.

Breathing responds instantly to emotions. When we are apprehensive, we breathe jerkily. We hold our breath if we are very afraid, and pain can make us gasp. Under stress some people breathe heavily and quickly, and hyperventilate. The sensations of hyperventilation are pins and needles in the fingers, numbness around the mouth, and a feeling of dizziness and sickness. Giving birth, even the most beautiful and satisfying birth, is a highly stressful activity, so it is understandable that many women over-breathe and hyperventilate when contractions are coming thick and fast.

During your pregnancy get to know your own breathing habits, noticing how your breathing changes with your emotions. If it is difficult to observe this, ask your partner to help. Are there any times when you tend to breathe arrhythmically, to hold your breath, or to over-breathe?

Tension in breathing usually stems from the shoulders. If you drop your shoulders, you will breathe more easily. Whenever you are aware of being under stress, breathe out, drop your shoulders, and relax. Your breathing will respond immediately and become rhythmic and even.

When you take time to relax, notice how you are breathing. Breathe smoothly and slowly so that it feels as if you are breathing down into your pelvis and touching your baby with your breath. When your breathing is relaxed like this, your baby often becomes active.

During labour, these long slow breaths will help at the onset and the end of every contraction. In early labour you may be able to breathe like this right through a contraction too. Sometimes it is possible to maintain this slow, steady breathing throughout the first stage – the longest part of labour when the cervix is dilating. But many women feel the need to breathe more quickly as contractions become more powerful and are closer together. If this is how it is for you, let your breathing speed up and at the same time *make it lighter*. Rapid deep breathing will result in hyperventilation (for more information see page 149). Rapid *light* breathing at the height of contractions can help you scale the peaks.

When contractions are at their strongest, it is impossible to move the abdominal wall or to feel anything in your pelvis other than their power. The tightening of longitudinal muscle fibres results in a lifting of the abdominal wall, because the contraction causes the top of the uterus, the fundus, to tilt forwards, so there is a great swelling that also presses against the diaphragm. From your diaphragm down, you feel as if you are all one huge contraction. Let your breathing "dance" above this and breathe through parted lips with the tip of your tongue resting against your lower teeth. Have sips of water or ice to suck in the spaces between contractions, so that your mouth does not get dry. Avoid huffing and puffing. The breath should be as light as a whisper. Then, as the contraction reaches its climax and starts to fade, you can form slow, full breaths again. It is important not to forget to do this. You and your baby will welcome the extra oxygen as each contraction finishes. And the slow breathing will help you relax completely in the trough between the great waves of contractions, so that you are refreshed and strong for the next one.

Breathing for labour is often taught in antenatal classes as a set of exercises, and sometimes these are very rigid and mechanical. It may be that when a woman is giving birth on alien territory, in a hospital where she is not sure what will happen to her, or what she will be allowed to do, such precise techniques are helpful as a distraction from pain and, above all, from an environment that she sees as threatening. The breathing exercises keep her busy and concentrated on something she can do to help herself. I have seen women with their eyes fixed on a crack in the ceiling breathing desperately, as if clinging to a safety rope above a precipice, mentally cut off from their surroundings, unable to hear what anyone is saying, completely out of touch with help that is being offered. When breathing is used like this, it becomes a barrier against the environment.

You will not need to use prelearned, rigid breathing if you are having your baby at home, or in the kind of out-of-hospital setting where your attendants are already friends, and where there is no need to fear intrusion.

When your cervix is wide open and your body ready for the baby to be pushed down, your breathing changes, often dramatically. There is an involuntarily held breath that starts as a catch in the throat. This is a sign that the baby is well on its journey and that you can help it out. While you can continue to breathe, you should do so. Do not attempt to hold your breath deliberately, as this forces the pace and causes unnecessary stress on your pelvic floor muscles and perineum.

Then, when you get an irresistible desire to push, drop your jaw, and *let yourself open up*, and breathe again as soon as the urge passes.

The baby's head will press deeper and deeper until you feel it bulging against your perineum like a grapefruit. You can put your hand down and touch it. From this point on, it is important to *breathe* your baby out, so that you push only when you cannot resist it. Your uterus will do the work for you. Breathing through your open, relaxed mouth, in long sighs, will help your perineum relax and unfold as the baby's head oozes through.

The head is born and rotates. You look down and have the first glimpse of your baby's profile. Then the shoulders slide through and, often in one quick movement, like a fish leaping, the whole body emerges, to reveal your slippery, warm, wriggling, wonderful baby.

TUNING IN TO YOUR BABY

When a woman does not wish professional caregivers to take over in childbirth, to manage her labour actively and make decisions without consulting her, it is important that she is in touch with her own feelings, with her body and the drama that is unfolding in it, and also with her baby. This little person is carried on the same waves of energy that sweep through her to the shores of life, sharing the experience with her.

"This child seems to understand laughter or, if we are all shouting and laughing, it starts kicking rhythmically. It touches with its feet anything placed over my abdomen. It feels like delicate exploring. There is an interval during which the baby must be locating the sensation, then a light kick in exactly the right spot."

The relationship with your baby starts long before your child is born, long before the very first contractions that herald labour. It has its tentative beginnings as soon as you are aware that you may have conceived, and ripens as you "listen" to your child's movements and conduct a two-way conversation with the world outside and the one within you. When you are in touch with your baby in the uterus, birth is only one stage in the development of a relationship that is already a reality.

A baby does not suddenly spring into action at birth. For some time before the event your baby has been a complex, coordinated human being who is already learning and communicating.

Babies react to touch very early, though at first this is merely a reflex response. By the time you are 12 weeks pregnant the baby is already kicking, but you do not feel it at this stage, because he or she is still too small. You usually feel movements for the first time between 17 and 20 weeks. They are like bubbles popping or minnows darting about. But even before that the baby can make complicated foot movements, twisting the foot round, curling and uncurling the toes, and "treading water".

At 16 weeks the baby reaches with tiny hands, feeling the water, and exploring the space around and the springy walls of the uterus.

Ultrasound reveals that babies often suck their thumbs, so pleasure from non-nutritive sucking is already well-established in the uterus. It assists the coordination of sucking and swallowing necessary for feeding. All the movements that the baby makes have the effect of toning its muscles, in the same way that regular exercise undertaken by adults results in muscular development and strengthening.

HOW YOUR BABY IS LYING

In the last few weeks of pregnancy you will probably be able to tell the position your baby is in by tracking the legs and trunk with your fingers. When your midwife or doctor palpates your uterus, he or she feels for the head first, but for you it is easier to start with the feet, which may be so clearly defined that you feel you could almost measure the baby for shoes. Starting from where you can find a vigorous little foot, pass your fingers along the legs to the baby's pointed bottom, and then feel down the long curve of the back.

If you are giving birth out of hospital, it will help to know if your baby is head down, if the head is engaged in your pelvis, and whether the baby's back is towards your front with the head tucked forwards on the chest. When this is the case, you can be increasingly confident that the birth will be straightforward.

When the baby is head down (in the vertex or cephalic position), you feel the kicking in the upper part of the uterus. When the baby's head is up, you feel the hard ball of the head under your ribs, although you may be deceived by a big baby who is lying head-down with its bottom positioned high under your ribs.

Once the head is engaged, your diaphragm can swing down more easily than before as you take a deep breath. When your bladder is full, the head may cause pressure against it so that you want to empty your bladder often, as in the first weeks of pregnancy. This is one sign that the head is deep in the pelvis. Another is an occasional buzzing and tingling in your vagina. The baby may be using your pelvic floor muscles as a trampoline, giving you short, sharp buzzing sensations like tiny electric shocks. These are a sign that the baby is in a very good position.

When the baby is curled into a ball with the back towards your front (in the anterior position), your navel protrudes and you can trace a firm, melon-shaped arc at the front. This is the baby's back. You will also be able to feel kicking at one side or the other under your ribs. Kicking occurs at the side opposite the baby's back.

If the baby is not yet anterior, you feel kicking all over your front, and there is a saucer-shaped dip around your navel. This suggests that the baby is posterior, with its back towards your spine. Strong contractions will be needed to turn the baby round into the ideal position for birth. Welcome them when they come, and prepare for a long first stage whilst your uterus does this work. You may have a backache labour, because the hard back of the baby's head is pressed into the small of your back. Discuss with your caregivers and birth partner how you are going to handle that.

Breech baby

If your baby is still not head down in the last weeks, you can try a pelvic tilt to shift the baby's bottom up out of your pelvis and enable him or her to somersault and turn head down. You will need to get your head lower than your pelvis, either by lying with your pelvis propped up over a couple of firm floor cushions or a beanbag with your head on the floor, or by supporting your pelvis on a low divan bed and leaning over the side of it. Lie turned towards your front rather than your back, as the baby will probably find it easier to move against your abdominal wall than against your spine. Make as much space as possible for your baby to move by ensuring that your knees are well apart and are not pressing against your abdomen. Once you are firmly fixed in position and have secure support, you can try moving your pelvis to encourage the baby to shift. Rolling and rocking movements are good. This is more likely to be effective at a time when you know the baby is awake and on the move. Although this may not be a posture you would choose for relaxation, once you are reasonably comfortable, relax and give long, slow, full breaths into your pelvis and release your abdominal muscles with each breath out.

More research needs to be done to discover whether this knee–chest position is really effective. Some babies somersault, but then turn back soon afterwards. Others refuse to budge at all. But, if your baby is still breech at the end of pregnancy, it is a manoeuvre worth trying for about 15 minutes, two or three times a day.

MAKING YOUR BIRTH PLAN

Discussing your ideas about the birth with whoever is going to attend you in labour helps you to focus your mind on what is most important to you, and enables your midwife or doctor to understand your needs.

In hospital, birth plans are often presented by anxious women, who are afraid that they will not be consulted about what is done to them during childbirth, to professionals who often feel very threatened by them. I have heard a birth plan described by an obstetrician as "a weapon used to manipulate the professionals" and by a psychotherapist as "a transitional object", like a security blanket.

One woman's birth plan
I should like to:

☐ Walk around for as long as possible.

☐ Stand or squat during contractions.

☐ Find out for myself which is the easiest and most comfortable position when pushing.

☐ Deliver the baby together with my husband, instead of having him as a tolerated onlooker.

☐ Have the comforting presence of one of my closest friends, who has two children herself.

☐ Have the same midwife present throughout: moreover a midwife who has given me antenatal care, whom I trust, and with whom I have a personal relationship.

☐ Receive no drugs.

" 'Birth plan?' said the doctor. 'What do you want?' I began to explain. 'What kind of things do you want to avoid, lovey?' she asked. I said I was not too keen on an episiotomy. She was absorbed in her own calculations. Suddenly she informed me that I was to be admitted straight away, as the baby had not grown in a fortnight. Labour might be induced that very afternoon. So much for my birth plan."

When you are having your baby out of hospital, a birth plan is a valuable element in the communication between you and your caregivers, part of the developing relationship with them. It ought to be like this in hospital too, but often isn't. Another problem with hospital birth plans is that, although you may be encouraged to make a plan, the person with whom you discuss what you want is unlikely to be with you right through labour, so a written birth plan becomes merely a set of orders handed over to a stranger. In the words of one irritated hospital administrator: "It happens in no other branch of medicine or other professional sphere that the client imposes crucial restrictions on the professional and tells him how to do his work." But it is quite clear with out-of-hospital birth that the discussion you have with your caregivers and the decisions to which you come are part of the vital process of getting to know each other, so that by the time you are in labour there is an understanding deeper than words.

Discuss with your midwife or doctor, or the small group of midwives who will look after you, the kind of care you would like, whom you want with you during labour, what your partner's role is likely to be, how you would prefer your newborn baby to be treated, and exactly what you are hoping for with this birth. Think about interventions you would prefer to avoid, and alternative ways of coping with difficulties. Discuss positions and movements you may want to choose, how you can get physical support for them, whether you want to use a bath or birth pool, and your thoughts about episiotomy, the clamping and cutting of the umbilical cord, and the conduct of the third stage. Then write down your decisions about the most important issues – if possible on just one sheet of paper. Ask your caregiver how it reads, and whether she or he is happy with it. Provide one copy to go with your records, and keep another yourself. If by any chance the person you are expecting to attend you in labour is not available, this birth plan will be invaluable and give a clear idea of your preferences.

" 'Are you going to make a birth plan?' the midwife asked. 'I think it is a good idea. We need to discuss ways in which you want to handle pain, so that I can help you. I think our ideas are much the same, but trust between us can't take the place of really knowing what you want.' "

YOUR BIRTH SPACE

You and your partner will want to create your own birth space. There is nothing especially modern about making a birth space, and it certainly isn't a fringe activity of educated middle-class couples. It is a kind of "nesting". Other mammals and birds line the nest with soft hay or moss, and in most human cultures the mother and those close to her prepare a special room. The Maori birth hut was actually called "the nesting house" and traditionally, in many parts of North and South America and Asia, women built their own birth huts, often close to water so that they could bathe after the baby was born. The space for receiving the baby was always constructed to be soft and warm. The Kwakiutl of British Columbia used to dig a shallow pit and line it with soft cedar bark, and the Pima of the American South West lined their birth pits with soft rabbit skin. Making one's own birth space is an important part of human culture, which is often neglected nowadays under the assumption that this space is designed to meet the needs of the professionals who conduct the birth, rather than the mother's, and that any personal touches are introduced merely as concessions to her.

Preparing your birth space
Things you may want to get together for an out-of-hospital birth:

- Beanbags or large floor cushions
- Camera
- Plenty of film, including fast film for night-time if you do not want to use a flash

- Sanitary pads, largest size
- Cotton pyjama tops, short nightdresses, or baggy T-shirts
- Face cloth
- Swimwear, so that your birth partner can go under the shower or into the bath or pool with you if you wish
- Socks for cold feet
- Nursing bras
- Two small real sponges, one to suck on while the other is in a bowl of cold water
- Small plant spray, filled with ice cold water to spray on your face
- Cracked ice to suck
- Cassettes and cassette player
- Candles, matches
- Eau de cologne
- Brush and comb, as well as hair-ribbons or clips to hold long hair away from your face and neck
- Essential oils
- Books, magazines
- Snacks for birth partner and midwife
- Honey, glucose drink, or herb teas
- Bendy straws
- Rolling pin with cloth tied over it, or wooden rolling massage animal, for back massage
- Painting, photographs, or sculpture to use as a visual focus
- Champagne or other celebration drink and food for after the birth

For birth away from home
- Spare can of petrol, in case your tank is empty
- Coins for the phone
- List of telephone numbers
- Baby clothes and clothes to wear going home

For birth at home
(Your midwife may provide some of these)
- Two buckets, one for sitting on, one for cleaning up
- New nail brush
- Bin liners
- Incontinence pads for sitting on – useful if you are leaking water or have a heavy show, as well as for afterwards so that bedding keeps clean

- Cleaning cloths
- Bottle of antiseptic
- Bowl for receiving placenta
- Portable lamp
- Large towels, one for you, one for baby, one for midwife
- Heavy plastic sheet over bed
- Tarpaulin or builders' plastic sheeting over carpet
- Extra heating if cold, fan if hot
- Frozen peas for cold compress
- Small hot-water bottle for hot compress
- Birth pool – or, if you want to soak in deep water and do not have a birth pool, Plasticine to plug the bath overflow

Your midwife's or doctor's equipment

Delivery pack; sphygmomanometer to take blood pressure; Pinard's stethoscope and/or sonic aid; urine-testing sticks; local anaesthetic and syringes; scissors; suture material, in case of damage to the perineum; mucus extractor, in case the baby's respiratory tract needs clearing; resuscitation equipment, in case the baby needs help to breathe; intravenous set and infusion, in case of bleeding; syntometrine and syringes, in case the uterus needs help to contract to expel the placenta.

If you are going into a GP unit or birth centre, take things with you that will help to make the room your personal space: a painting, photographs, a plant, a mobile perhaps. If you are giving birth at home, you may want to choose a room that is small, dark, and private. But the birthplace does not have to be the bedroom, although a big double bed is lovely if there is room in it for the whole family just after the birth. If you have a garden, you may want to be outside for a time, and squat holding on to a tree when contractions come. You may want to use water – with the bath, shower, jacuzzi, or a special birth pool. (There are details of how to hire a pool on page 196.) If so, do you want your partner to be in the water with you or not? You may feel differently when you are in labour, but at least you can plan ahead for a range of possibilities and experiment with different positions and movements in water.

Using a birth pool

The ideal room for a birth pool is probably on the ground floor, with one door opening out on to a garden and another on to a darkened, comfortable room where you can escape all the pressures of the outside world and sink

"If you are tired and aching, the first thing you want to do is have a bath. That's why I have hired a birth pool."

Opposite *Being in water eases pain, and enables you to move more freely and to explore positions in which your pelvis is at its widest, such as wide-open kneeling.*

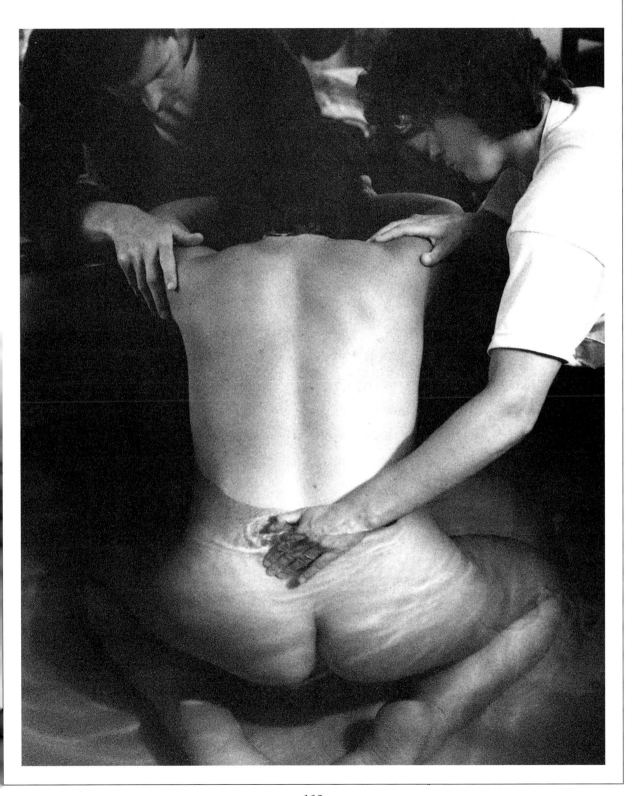

deeply into your own sensations. If it is warm weather, you can then labour part of the time in the fresh air, and withdraw to your womb-like room or float peacefully in the pool the rest of the time. The important thing is to be free to move between these different environments and not feel committed to water birth come what may.

If you want to have the birth pool in an upstairs room and the floor is wooden, check with the people from whom you are hiring it or a friendly builder that the floor can take its weight when it is filled with water. This will be about one tonne.

There are two hoses with the pool. One has attachments to connect it securely to the taps. Allow a good hour to fill the pool. The second enables you to run off water, so that you can feed in fresh hot water through the other hose or empty the pool. To avoid having hosepipes snaking all over the place, the pool is best located not far from a sink or bath. Think about where you are going to let the waste water run – perhaps straight into a drain or garden. A pool equipped with an electric pump can be emptied rapidly. It helps to have an efficient domestic hot water supply. If necessary, turn up the thermostat on the immersion heater, but be very careful if you have other children in the house. Some pools have heaters similar to those used in aquaria. Although they maintain the water at a comfortable temperature, they are not powerful enough to heat it from cold, and you may not like the idea of having a heater in the pool when you are in it. The pool should have a plastic cover that, even without a heater, retains heat well, so that once filled the pool will stay warm for eight to ten hours.

Set the pool up about ten days before the baby is due and use it for relaxation and centering down into positive thoughts about birth. It helps to alleviate late-pregnancy backache, and feels good if you have clusters of painful Braxton-Hicks contractions or a long lead into labour. Empty the pool every 24 hours or so, and refill with clean water. It is usually not difficult to keep the water clean. A plastic sieve can be used to scoop any debris out of the water.

The water does not need to be very warm. Just around blood temperature is right, though you will want the air around the pool to be warm so that after the birth the baby does not lose heat rapidly and you can cuddle her while still sitting in the water. In the second stage you may get very hot, and it feels good if the water is cool. Cooler water helps you mobilize your energy to push the baby out and stimulates the urge to bear down.

At birth, lift your baby so that at least her head is free of the water. Two babies have died by being kept under water as if they were fish, not human beings. The important thing is that there are loving arms to welcome the baby. At birth the child slips out of your body, feels the smooth, liquid touch of water, and then, as she takes the first breath of air and her lungs inflate, is welcomed with a passionate, tender and exultant embrace. It is all part of a sequence that reaches its climax when a baby is held in her mother's arms and gazes into her eyes for the very first time.

Creating comfort and the right atmosphere

When you are on dry land, have a stool or beanbag, or a bucket with a rolled towel around the rim, ready to support you in a squatting position. A lunge position with the forward knee bent is easily adopted on the stairs, or with one foot up on a small stool – such as the kind a child uses to reach the lavatory – or on a few encyclopedias. The banisters or bathroom towel rail may be of the right height to provide a good squatting bar. In rural Africa women often kneel or squat, holding the house post that supports the roof. When my first baby was born, I spontaneously squatted grasping the heavy, bulbous legs of a Victorian table. It was a hideous table, but good and solid, and felt just right.

With your partner, think what kind of lighting would be best. Lamps that can be dimmed are pleasant. Would you like candles? If your birth attendant wants a bright light on your perineum to see exactly what is happening, how can this be arranged? On a bright day you may like the room flooded with sunlight, or prefer a soft glow through curtains or blinds.

Consider how you will warm and air the room too. You will want to be comfortably warm in labour. In winter you may like to give birth on a hearthrug or a couch in front of the flickering flames of a guarded open fire, or in summer in a room opening on to the garden. You may feel very hot in the second stage and want to have a window wide open or an electric fan available. The baby is emerging from a hot-house atmosphere inside your body, and needs to be born into warm air, so a fan heater that can be switched on as the birth approaches is a good idea.

Think together about the things around you that you will find comforting, and that will enhance your positive visualization of what is happening in your body. If you would like background music, you can plan this together, and it will help if you practise relaxation whilst playing this music, so that you associate it with complete release of mind and body. The sounds you choose don't have to be music. You could record the dawn chorus of bird song if you wish, or waves breaking on the shore. One of my own babies was born as a blackbird sang in the apple tree outside my bedroom window. It was an enormously reassuring, happy sound, and I felt that nature was conspiring with me to make the birth beautiful for all of us.

For good smells there is a wide range of aromatherapy oils to choose from, and you may like to have scented candles, bunches of lavender, or flowers in the room. When my fourth baby was born, my bedroom was full of bowls of hyacinths, and I always associate the heady scent of hyacinths with that particular birth.

IMAGES OF BIRTH

An important part of your preparation for birth is nothing to do with exercises or information: it is simply to daydream.

When you relax and focus on positive sensory images of birth, you open up possibilities for a richer and deeper experience. These images should always be realistic in the sense that they are based on acknowledgement that labour is stressful, that the power of the uterus is awesome, that when the cervix is opening to its full extent it is usually painful, and that when the baby's head is in your vagina there is an incredible sensation of pressure. You can anticipate, acknowledge, and affirm all these sensations in a positive way.

The words you use are vital elements in these anticipatory fantasies. Language is never neutral. It presents a view of the world. Most of the words we have about pregnancy and birth are not only man-made but also medical. A woman is an "elderly primigravida" or "high risk". She has "an untried pelvis". Doctors' names are attached to processes in women's bodies as if these medical men had somehow invented them. The contractions she experiences in late pregnancy are known as "Braxton-Hicks". Dilatation of the cervix must follow the "Friedman curve". To use medical language is to impose on yourself a medical view of birth. Sometimes these medical terms are the only words available, so we need to translate them into women's language, and create words that have immediate meaning for us in terms of our own feelings and the ways in which we can express ourselves through our bodies.

Your pelvis, for example, is not just an anatomical structure, a piece of architecture through which the fetus is pushed. As you think of it, explore metaphors and other images that enable you to have a more dynamic view of it. When you rock your pelvis with your baby nestled inside, it is like a cradle. As you sing, hum, or chant, it becomes a resonator. Sometimes it may feel more like a mysterious cave, or like a treasure chest that holds the power of the uterus. In a woman's pelvis the ebb and flow of menstrual tides take place and, when the time is right, the full drama of birth is enacted. You can create your own images. You need not use second-hand ones.

These anticipatory fantasies derived from sensory experience need not all be visual. They can be auditory, for example, based on passages from music and ideas of cadence, harmony, rhythm, and being in tune with your body.

They can be tactile too. A feeling of the baby moving inside you is one of intense and often surprising touch. As the uterus contracts and your baby moves down to enter the world, you feel intense pressure, your waters may break with a soft splash, and you are aware of your baby's firm head sliding down – solid and rounded as a grapefruit – and of quivering, throbbing heat as the head crowns. As it slips forwards and you reach down to feel it, your fingers touch soft, wet hair, and you are astonished at the otherness of this little creature who has for so long been a part of yourself but is now being born from your body.

Kinetic images may come to mind too. Your breathing dances, you get into the swing of contractions, swimming over each as it rises in crescendo, or breasting it like a great ocean wave. You float, you ride, you ski down the mountain slopes, you leap into the void. I shall never forget an Israeli woman who, as each contraction swelled up, proclaimed: "Gates of Jerusalem, open for me!" And for her this was the intense image that most accurately expressed the sense of her body opening wide as she gave birth.

The imagery that is likely to be helpful to you will include active verbs of opening, releasing, spreading, unfolding, and fanning out. As contractions sweep through you, concepts that suggest power, energy, strength, and, perhaps, storm and even whirlwind suddenly make sense, along with wave and water fantasies – verbs such as stream, pool, flood, gush, flow, and cascade. And all over the world, in many different cultures, women use visual images of fruit ripening and of the baby's head like a hard bud in the centre of a flower's unfurling petals.

As you read about birth, and whenever you take time to relax and enjoy anticipatory fantasies, create your own images and dreams that will give positive meaning to all the sensations of labour. Doing this will help you to savour fully an adventure that can be among the most thrilling, intense and satisfying experiences of your life.

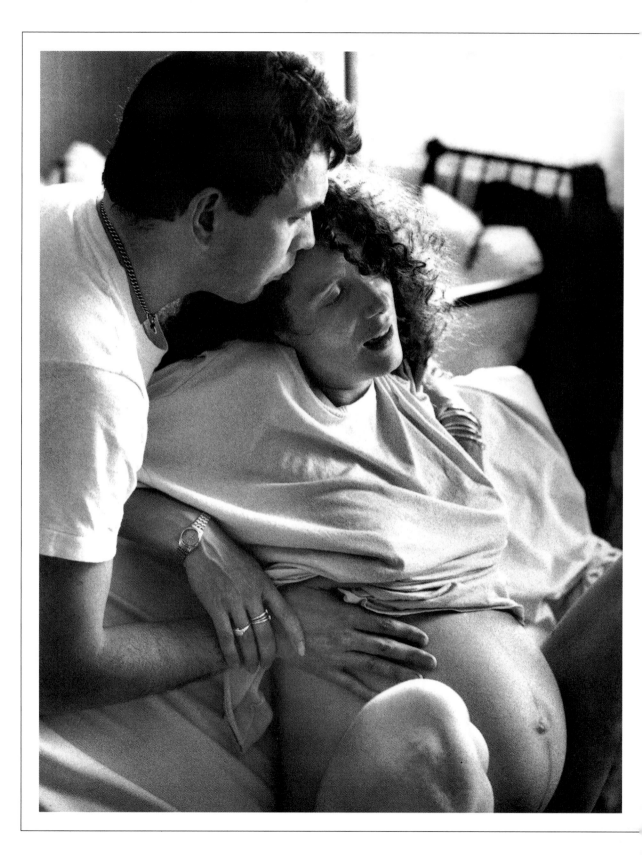

7

Your Birth Partner

Sharing the experience of childbirth with someone who is close to you helps give you strength and confidence. When you have a baby at home this person is usually your sexual partner because birth occurs quite naturally as a part of the flow of your relationship. When birth is in a GP unit or birth centre, you may want your sexual partner with you as this special person, or you may want someone else – an intimate friend or relative.

MALE ANXIETIES ABOUT BIRTH

In the past men distanced themselves from birth, both its physiological and emotional aspects. It was not "manly" to do anything else. They strode the hospital corridors while their wives laboured. They crouched smoking in the fathers' waiting room. They went to a pub and drank themselves silly to anaesthetize their fears. Or they tried to concentrate on work as if nothing important was happening. They denied the strength of their own anxiety. It was as if a script was already written for them and they had to accept their allotted roles. Men lost out as well as women. The taboo on tenderness, of which this was one example, meant that they were expected to be strong to shoulder burdens, to earn money to support their wives and children, and to protect territory, but were not allowed to be aware of the intricacies of human emotion or the subtleties of relationships. If they were, they had to put on an act and pretend that they were tough and strong. The role stereotype was basically ape-like, not human.

"Chris was looking at the baby with his complete attention, his face transfigured with happiness and wonder. He looked like a small child seeing something more wonderful than he had ever seen before."

In the span of 30 years, fathers' involvement in childbirth in Western culture, novel in the 60s, has come to be accepted as normal. Maybe the idea of fathers at birth contained the seed of "the new man", the male personality who is not grabbing, fighting, and crude, but who can be nurturing and tender. But, in spite of many fathers now attending the births of their babies, this new man is a much heralded but still rare creature – a new and endangered species in a rough, tough world. Yet each time a woman gives birth and a man has the opportunity to share the experience and to grow in understanding, there is at least a chance that not only a baby but a man with a deeper awareness and sensitivity will be born.

On the other hand it is easy to be over-optimistic about the changes that can be brought about when fathers are involved in childbirth in hospital. A concerned, caring father can help with communication and give his partner strong emotional support. But hospitals are organized so that even the most determined man may go along with the system all too easily and fail to give the support a woman needs.

When fathers began to be at births back in the 60s, their presence was at first resisted by many doctors and midwives, who felt that their territory was threatened. But within a few years fathers came to be warmly welcomed, as staff realized that most of them turned into subordinate, well-behaved members of the birth "team", who could be relied upon to help control the woman's behaviour, keep her calm, and make her "see reason" when staff wished to intervene against her wishes.*

Men still often feel out of place in hospital childbirth, and do everything they can to maintain good relations with staff, to be polite and compliant, and to prevent the woman "making a fuss" or drawing attention to herself. They go into hospital with the firm purpose of giving labour support, but many are cowed into submission by the whole atmosphere of the unit and by the evident authority of the senior men who are in charge. Fathers often feel violent emotions welling up inside them because of how their partners are being treated, yet are conditioned by their education to block the expression of disturbing feelings, and to be obedient team members. In this state of mind they are inclined to play the hospital game, to collude with the medical system, and women are left feeling isolated and abandoned.

Most obstetricians are men, and it is unlikely that this has occurred by chance. They want to control women in the most essentially female activity of giving birth. So they invent machinery to enable them to do this more effectively. It is almost a truism to say that men like machines, enjoy tinkering with them, and rely on them more than women. It *is* only a truism, because it is usually women who operate and understand the idiosyncrasies of electric irons and kettles, vacuum cleaners, washing machines, dishwashers, mixers, sewing machines, typewriters, and wordprocessors. Because men are accustomed to being in control of women, obstetricians manage childbirth – or at least achieve a semblance of management – with electronic equipment. Prospective fathers are often reassured when they see the technology available in the modern hospital, whereas their female partners tend to be disturbed by it. Of course there are some men who are made equally anxious by all this high-tech gear, just as there are women who breathe a sigh of relief and believe that nothing can go wrong if it is to hand. But they are probably in the minority.

"We felt strongly that our child should emerge into her father's arms and share that first breath of life in the intimate bond of the family."

Fathers' sharing in the birth experience can be the stimulus for men's freedom to nurture, and a sign of changing relationships between men and women. In the same way, women's freedom to give birth at home is a political decision, an assertion of our determination to reclaim the experience of birth. Birth at home is about changing society.

THE DEEPER MEANINGS OF BIRTH

Sharing the experience of birth can be a peak event in a loving relationship, something that is never forgotten. Rahima Baldwin, who helps run the Dearborn Garden of Life Birth Center, where half the parents are Arab, speaks movingly of "the profound moment when the father whispers the *al-adhan*, or call to prayer," to his newborn child. Men who were not at all sure at first that they wanted to be present say afterwards: "I wouldn't have missed it for the world." For many it is as if suddenly they are face to face with life's real meaning, and a power even more overwhelming than sexual desire.

When women are asked afterwards what their partners did that helped, they often say: "It was just that he was *there*." Being present *in the moment*, not distracting or distracted, but right there *with her*, is the essence of being a birth partner. It is nothing to do with coaching the woman, as the father's role is often described in North American childbirth education. It is not a matter of complicated techniques, but of giving her complete and focused concentration.

It is possible to be physically present with a woman in labour and not be there at all. I remember accompanying one couple having a hospital birth for whom the event was a truce in a long-drawn-out battle. The husband, who was a doctor, brought his transistor radio into the delivery room and, as his wife was pushing the baby out, he switched on the news and listened to it intently, until I suggested that this was the wrong time and place for it and asked him to get behind her to support her head and shoulders. It may be that delivery rooms and women in the second stage were so commonplace for him that he did not see any need to be emotionally involved. Or he may have been trying to punish his wife. Or perhaps he was trying to protect himself from overwhelming emotion, and was frightened that he might actually feel too much.

Your birth partner should prepare with you for the birth, not just be called in when you start labour. He or she should be someone who understands your needs and knows exactly when it is appropriate to give help and when to stand back.

Men are often poorly prepared for the experience of childbirth. A study of what fathers actually did when they had planned to act as "labour coaches" in a Canadian hospital revealed that they spent a lot of time trying to hide their feelings and worrying that they were not being useful.* Though most had attended childbirth classes, they were not able to help in the way they had expected, and their emotions proved very different from those anticipated. The hospital environment often inhibits a birth partner from giving a woman full support and puts him under great stress. He feels surrounded by experts, is scared of doing the wrong thing and, if the woman becomes distressed as labour progresses, he becomes increasingly anxious. Birth in an out-of-hospital setting provides an environment in which the birth partner can also be *himself*. He doesn't feel that he has to put on an act.

"Nicholas was where I needed him about ten seconds before I knew where that was! I felt supported, but not pushed, by all three of them."

"Philip fixed me with his eyes gently and kindly, yet insistently. He never allowed me to sink into the pain. Eye contact and simultaneous breathing with him got me through the contractions."

"The birth was made much easier by being in comfortable, familiar and planned surroundings, and having midwives who were our friends, rather than the staff of an institution, visiting our own home and helping us through a difficult but exciting and joyful time."
A father

FEELINGS ABOUT BIRTH

Anyone who is present at a birth brings to it their own emotions, their own expectations, their fear and hope, and their love. As a baby is born, there is not only the mother's birth passion, but the often intense emotions of all others involved. This is why emotional preparation is vital. Childbirth education is not just a matter of learning what happens and knowing how to help. It should be a process that leads to greater self-awareness.

Whether your birth partner is your sexual partner or some other person, it is important to talk together about your feelings beforehand.

☐ What is most important to you about the birth?

☐ What do you want of your birth partner?

☐ How does your birth partner feel about this?

☐ What kind of help will your partner need to give?

☐ How does your partner feel about this?

Emotions about birth are often complex and powerful. You can explore feelings further by each going on to finish the statement, "When I think about the birth, I feel . . . " Listen to each other without judgement and, if some of these emotions turn out to be threatening, do not try to change them or protest that there is no need to feel like this. Just accept them.

Can you remember your first contact with birth as a child? As I talk with couples, I find that earliest memories are often negative. Adults may recall bewilderment and pain when their mother was whisked off to hospital, they were left without her, and then presented with a baby who replaced them. They may also remember hushed, pitying voices as "female problems" were discussed, or an aunt's "bad time" as women talked in shocked whispers about the number of stitches she had. All these experiences must colour our view of birth, even if only to make us determined to do things differently.

Many men are not sure that they can handle seeing the woman they love in pain, or cope with being close to the sheer physicality of birth. If you have seen a birth film, talk about your feelings as you watched it too. Viewing a film is very different from being fully involved in a birth. With a film you are merely a spectator, and there is nothing you can do about it. In a birth you are *needed* and caught up in the yearning and excitement. It is the difference between watching a film of surfers on Bondi Beach and actually being there and riding the waves yourself.

Talking about how your partner has felt in the past when you have been in pain, or were ill or especially vulnerable, can also help deepen your understanding of each other. What did you want then? The pain of birth is functional, creative, positive. It is pain with a purpose. In an intimate atmosphere the physicality of birth can be close to that of love-making. The swelling uterus straining against the abdominal wall, the woman's quickened breathing, her damp skin and hair and shining eyes, the astonishing urge to push, and the energy that pours through her, the grunts and moans as she presses the baby down, the bulging perineum, the top of the baby's head like a wrinkled walnut in her vagina, and then oozing through – all these elements in birth are *sexual* when they are not made medical in the context of hospital care.

Women often dream more during pregnancy. Dreams that were previously grey turn technicoloured. Men may dream too, and their dreams may express hopes and anxieties about birth. Sometimes there is fear of losing the woman, of the baby being abnormal, or of not being able to measure up to what is required of them. While I am not suggesting that you go into lengthy dream analysis, dreams can often provide clues to the problems we are trying to sort out in our lives and the challenges we face. It helps just to realize this and to say, "Yes, I am worried about it," and to think whether there is some positive action that you can take to deal with the challenge. Even when there is nothing practical to be done, simple acknowledgement of fear often enables you to handle it.

A WOMAN FRIEND

Sometimes a man wants to be present but feels that he cannot take entire responsibility for giving emotional support. Then having another person as well, a woman who understands birth, may be a good idea. In North America this person may be called a "professional labor assistant" or a "doula", a Greek word meaning "the woman who serves" and in France a "monitrice", which means "the woman who watches and is aware". When a couple are together, the task is not to take over, but to support them both. As one labor assistant put it: "I am there to help a woman, just like her mother or father was when she learned to ride a bicycle. During birth I am like the parent who held on to the back of the bicycle until the rider had some experience and felt safe and turned around to see that she had been riding on her own for quite some time."*

The notion that a woman can have only one companion with her, and that this must be the baby's father, stems from the time in the late 60s when fathers were first allowed in delivery rooms, and women were told that no one else could possibly come because there was no room. Over and over again senior midwives and doctors explained to couples, "Our hospital wasn't designed for this," and they often went on to say, "We have the midwife and her assistant and the doctor and the medical students, so there just isn't space." Notices were often put up by delivery suite doors: "No admission. Fathers only." This was hard on single mothers and on any woman who wanted a woman friend with her instead of a man.

Now in many countries the father's presence is unquestioned. But in ritualizing the attendance of fathers and making it almost mandatory, women are denied the right to choose another person, or perhaps several people with different qualities to offer. It is only in a home setting that these decisions can be made freely; and it is important that they *are* made, and that a reluctant or anxious father does not hang around simply because he lives there and everyone assumes that he is the obvious birth partner.

BEING A BIRTH PARTNER

"I didn't need him to do anything. I didn't want to be told what to do. Being able to rely on him, knowing he wouldn't leave me, seeing him there smiling as I came out of every contraction, that was what I needed."

Your birth partner is someone who is an anchor in a stormy sea. Being able to remain calmly confident is the single most important quality needed. There are many ways of giving comfort when the going gets tough and of refreshing you if you feel so tired that you wish it was all over. You will learn about these skills in childbirth classes and have a chance to rehearse them and find out which are likely to suit you best. When you do this in a group with other couples, you can learn a great deal from each other and can also share ideas.

It often helps for your birth partner to use words and phrases that were used in the childbirth classes – those that held most meaning for you. They can be very simple, such as "open", "release", "lovely", or "good", or repeated phrases, such as "let it flow", "you are strong", "you are doing really well", "that's another one gone", or "we're getting there". But this must be done with discretion. No one wants to be hectored or cajoled in labour. If help is offered without empathy, it can seem as if the other person is taking over, and a woman may think: "Who's having this baby, you or me?" So keep words to the minimum.

"When I was in transition, I said 'I'm bloody well not doing this again,' and he reminded me: 'You must be nearly fully dilated. It won't be long now! Take one contraction at a time.' When I did that, the pain was suddenly manageable."

I have found myself in the role of birth partner in countries where I have been studying women's experiences of birth and have not spoken the language. All I needed to do was know a few words, such as "softly", "breathe", "gently", "open wide", and "beautiful", with which to reach out to a woman, and these have been enough to give strong birth support. I aim to be beside a woman, not *over* her but *with* her. Separated by culture, education, and language, we yet encounter each other as sisters.

In the same way, whatever techniques birth partners acquire, however much they learn, the essence of what they give to the woman in birth is that they are her lovers and friends, not assistants to the midwife, barefoot doctors, or labour "coaches".

TOUCH, MASSAGE, AND HOLDING

"It was good having him to squeeze tight, and I knew he wouldn't mind how hard I squeezed. With anyone else I would have felt bound to apologize, but I just clung on to him."

When you feel tossed and lost and broken by fierce contractions coming in quick succession, being held firmly helps you feel safe. Your partner's hand stroking lightly or massaging you deeply can relieve pain even when it is very threatening, depending on where and how the touch is given. Any kind of physical contact from a person whom you trust can, if given with discretion and sensitivity, help you relax in a situation of stress. One strong benefit of not being in an alien environment is that your partner is unlikely to feel inhibited in giving you physical support and caring for you freely through touch.

During pregnancy you can explore together ways of touching and holding, so that just a look or gesture from you will indicate to your birth partner when and where you want to feel the reassurance and energy that is given by a loved hand.

Before you practise, prepare some massage oil – vegetable oil or nut oil lightly scented with any essential oil that you find relaxing. Then strip down to your underclothes and settle in a warm, comfortable place, well supported by pillows.

Stroking
Your partner can make contact with the baby by stroking your abdomen lightly. You will notice that this touch needs to be made with really relaxed, warm hands. So it is worth spending a few minutes loosening hands before starting by shaking them vigorously from the wrists as if flicking water from the finger-tips. For all massage, your partner's shoulders need to be loose too. If they are tight, tension is conveyed down the arm into the hand and can even cause pain.

Slow, light stroking over the lower abdomen can feel good in labour, especially before 5 cm dilatation of the cervix. If your partner is slightly to one side of you, an oiled hand can be drawn from underneath the far curve of your abdomen in an arc down over the place where your cervix is dilating, and then up again over the nearer side, followed by the other hand

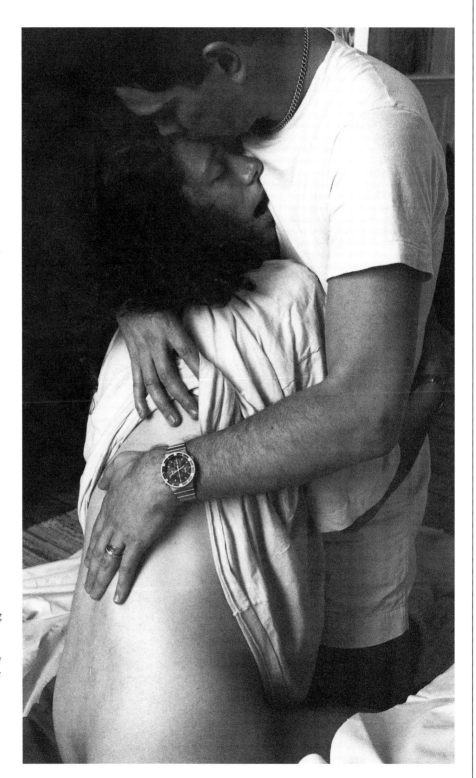

When contractions are coming every two or three minutes a woman often feels that she needs an anchor in the stormy sea of labour, and wants to be upright and firmly held.

using a similar smooth movement in the same direction. The resulting light finger-tip massage seems to be stroking the baby's head.

Shoulder massage

The tension that results in over-breathing and hyperventilation starts in the shoulders, and a shoulder massage helps you loosen these muscles. Your partner is behind you, fingers resting on your shoulders, and massages firmly with thumbs in the valleys either side of your spine. Then try moving the thumbs slowly and firmly in a circular motion over your shoulder blades.

Back massage

Long, slow, sweeping movements with the hands down either side of your spine can help you relax completely between contractions, so that you do not carry over tension from one contraction to another. First the hands rest on the shoulders. Then one hand is moved firmly, without haste, sweeping down your back. When this hand reaches your bottom, the other hand joins in the movement, and slowly sweeps down the other side, as the first hand is replaced on your shoulder, and so on. Your partner will need to have a relaxed body to do this easily, as this massage is only satisfying when he literally gets into the rhythmic swing of it.

When there is back pain, it is usually most concentrated at the sacrum, the big bone where your pelvis is attached to your spine, or to one side of this. Pain in this region is helped by very firm circular massage from the heel of the palm with the other hand resting over it, so that pressure comes from the weight of your partner's back down the shoulders and arms into the hands. When you practise this, try the effect of your partner being at different angles to your body, because the pressure you feel will be different depending on whether it is exerted in an upward or downward direction. It may be most effective when your partner is near your shoulders, so that this pressure is exerted downwards on your sacro-lumbar ligaments.

Foot massage

Your partner holds your feet in his or her lap and first squeezes your foot above and below, your calf muscles front and back, and then massages the soles of your feet with the thumbs. This can be done between strong contractions. As the next contraction builds up, the hands are stilled, and firm thumb pressure is exerted just below the big toe of each foot, slightly in towards the next toe. If you experiment with this, you will find a spot in which strong pressure produces a slight buzzing sensation. It is an acupressure (shiatsu) pain-prevention point.

"My midwife was warm, loving, and calm. She massaged my feet and kept encouraging me. I looked into Nick's eyes and saw the love he has for me. This kept me going through a 36-hour labour."

Giving counter-pressure

You may appreciate firm counter-pressure rather than moving touch. So much is happening inside you that any movement may be distracting and break your concentration. Counter-pressure is particularly effective for low back pain if strong hands rest one on top of the other over exactly the right spot, and your partner's weight is allowed to flow down the arms. As the baby presses lower, pressure like this may feel good over your buttocks.

Kneading

Deep massage into the flesh and underlying muscles can help you cope with sensations which might otherwise seem preposterous and threatening. As the baby's head presses against your rectum and anus, it may feel as if you are about to empty your bowels. Then, as the head fans out all the tissues, it feels like a huge ball just behind your anus. To help you relax your buttock and pelvic floor muscles, your partner can knead your buttocks using thumbs or thumbs and fingers as if kneading bread dough.

Holding

Holding is helpful not only for physical support in upright positions, but when you just need to know that someone is *there*, focused entirely on you, or when you want to be steadied and anchored.

Some good holding positions with which you and your birth partner can experiment are: supporting the back of your shoulders; encircling a wrist; grasping your feet; holding the bony ridge of your pelvis on either side; and cradling your head with a hand on each side or one hand cupped over the back of your head. Your partner should stay quite still, feeling and sharing the power that is sweeping through your body.

You can find much more about touch, massage, and holding in my book *Pregnancy and Childbirth*, details of which are on page 200.

MOVING AROUND

When you are in labour, it will help if you have already explored with your birth partner movements and positions you are most likely to find comfortable, bearing in mind as you do so that upright positions will enable your uterus to contract freely and the baby's head to rotate and descend. One great advantage of home birth is that you will already know exactly what you can use for comfort and physical support – walls, window ledges, and furniture – and you don't have to use any special apparatus such as a squatting bar or birth chair.

Experiment with the following movements and positions together:

☐ Walk about and then, as you imagine a contraction, lean forwards on to your partner with your legs well apart and knees unlocked. Try this facing your partner, behind him, and at his side. Experiment with him standing with his back against the wall for support. Then try it with him sitting on a chair or table.

☐ Find out in which of these positions that you have just practised your partner can rub your back easily. Walk around again, and this time imagine contractions coming with low backache. Your partner massages you firmly in the small of your back where your pelvis joins your spine. Massage is best done at one side or both sides of the spine, not right on it, and using the heel of the palm rather than the fingers or flat of the hand.

☐ Walk again and when an imaginary contraction starts, lean forwards on to a wall in any way that is comfortable for you. Your partner massages you as you stand in this position.

☐ Sit facing the back of an upright chair, leaning over a pillow on the back of the chair, with your shoulders rounded, feet flat on the floor. Your partner can massage your back in this position.

☐ Now turn so that you sit on the chair in the conventional way. Your partner kneels in front of you and you lean over him.

There are many other positions and movements you can explore, using your partner for support or being massaged by him, or sometimes both at once. Other positions to try are: kneeling with legs wide apart, leaning forwards with your head on a pillow on a chair in front of you; kneeling upright; half-kneeling, half-squatting, with one foot flat on the floor; an all-fours position; and squatting, leaning forwards with your hands on the floor. In many of these positions you may also welcome additional physical support from your birth partner.

Once you feel confident being supported by your partner in a range of positions, explore movements you may want to make. With some of these you may like your partner to be still. With others it feels best if your partner moves with you in the same rhythm.

☐ Rock your pelvis on all fours while your partner rests a hand at either side of your pelvis.

☐ Squat, leaning forwards and holding on to your partner, and then rock your pelvis to and fro.

☐ Try kneeling and leaning over your partner, who is on all fours in front of you, and rock your pelvis in this position.

When the second stage of labour starts and you are pushing the baby out, you don't have to go to bed unless you want to. You may have the ideal bed – a four-poster – and be able to squat holding on to one of the posts, or a bed with a solid headboard which you can grasp as you kneel facing it. If you are using a bed, it is best if the mattress is firm. But it may feel better to be on a clean sheet on the floor. Explore with your partner some of the positions you may want to use:

☐ Stand with your partner behind you holding your elbows, wrists, or hands, whichever is most comfortable. If he is taller than you, he should keep a straight back, bending his knees slightly.

☐ Stand in front of and facing your partner, with your hands clasped around his neck.

☐ With your partner sitting behind you, sit upright between his legs, with your knees drawn up and legs well apart. Use pillows as necessary for extra support for you both.

With all your preparations together, however, you will need to be flexible so that you can do whatever feels right at the time of birth, even if it is not what you planned. It is important for a birth partner to know when to be silent, when to give you your own space, when not to intrude and when to let you flow with the labour. The power of birth is like the strength of water cascading in a mighty rush down the hillside. It is the power of seas and tides, the power of mountains moving. There is no way of ignoring it. You cannot fight it. No amount of technique can enable you to be in control of it as you might be in control of a car or a computer. Your birth partner should aim not to manage, conduct, or coach you through this experience, but rather to give you strength and confidence as you allow your body to open and your baby to press through it to life.

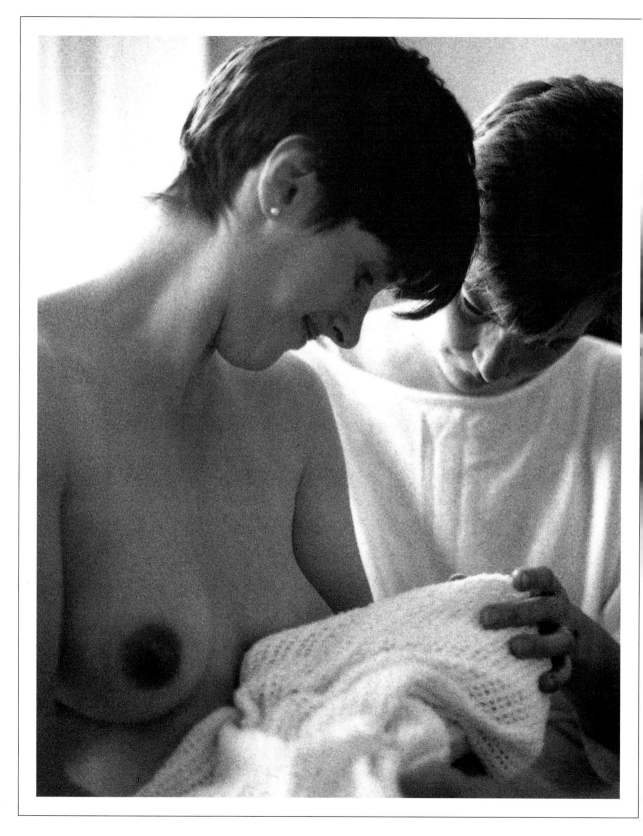

8

Sharing the Experience

Having a strong support group, sharing the experience of pregnancy, swapping your accounts of interviews with obstetricians, of hospital visits, and previous labours, and dealing with the medical system can help you discover what your rights are and learn effective strategies. During labour too you may want to have close friends or family with you. They can increase your confidence and give a great deal of comfort.

THE NEED FOR SUPPORT

When you plan a birth outside hospital, it helps to have a network of supporters – other couples and women – with whom you can share experiences, develop effective strategies for coping, and work together towards change. You will probably find other such like-minded people in your antenatal class, among your midwife's other clients, and in childbirth organizations (see those listed on page 196). If you are having a baby in an alternative birth centre, you will be able to talk to newly delivered women and their partners over a cup of tea in the kitchen when you visit, and will soon find that you are part of a group of prospective and new parents who support the birth centre. In the same way the groups formed to defend GP units that are threatened with closure, in countries where the policy is one of centralization, are strongly cohesive and militant in a very positive, celebratory way, and you will make new friends and discover many others who think as you do.

In most countries a woman who wants a home birth tends to be isolated, has to fight a lonely battle, and may be treated by doctors as if she is suffering from severe emotional problems. Sometimes a hospital obstetrician has gone so far as to threaten a woman with psychiatric detention or with having her newborn baby confiscated because of her "irresponsibility". It is too much to expect a woman to be able to handle this hostility alone. In her book, *Midwives and Medical Men*, Jean Donnison says of women seeking home birth that they need "the patience of Job, the courage of Joan of Arc, and the political skill of a Metternich".*

Support from other women

Traditionally a woman in childbirth has always had other women helping her. As well as the midwife, there were friends, family members, and neighbours who gave emotional and practical support. In 1658 Ralph Josselin recorded in his diary that his wife's labour had been so quick that, besides the midwife and nurse (for the baby), "only two or three women more got to her but God supplied all, young Mrs Harlakenden got up to us very speedily, and some others".*

Other women still give support to women in childbirth in most Third World countries. When anthropologists are present at a birth, it is often quite difficult for them to find out who exactly the midwife is, because she is one of a group of women helpers engaged in a task within a non-medical context. Childbirth is like bread-baking, laundering, or cheese-making – activities that involve a community of women working together. In our own

"We were sure that we didn't want to have our child come into a group of strangers, but rather into the loving circle of family and friends in a familiar setting."

"I'd never had that feeling so strongly before, of women sharing a process they understood and in complete harmony with each other. It was like a dance in which you all hear the same music and move accordingly, without having to talk about it."

past, and cross-culturally, every adult woman was expected to know what to do in childbirth and how to help other women. She might have a recipe for a strengthening broth to be taken during labour, have herbs to stimulate the uterus, or a lodestone or charm to help the birth go well.

Throughout Europe in medieval times, when a woman started labour, she called on other women in the neighbourhood, who came bringing food to sustain them all during the labour and for celebration after the birth, and plenty of strong drink. Men were turned out of the house as women took over. These women would later testify at the baptism of the child, and were known as God sibs, literally "sisters in God". Men must have resented this female takeover, and in English the words "God sib" gradually became changed in male usage to "gossip".

In pioneer times in North America women relied heavily on what was known in Canada as "turn-about" help. It carried on the old European tradition but with a new urgency, since many of them were in isolated communities. Women had to be able to heal illness, mend bones, comfort the dying, and help one another in childbirth. When a baby was on the way, they made each other baby clothes and sewed beautiful bed quilts and then, when labour started, cooked meals, did the housework, took over the woman's other duties, such as milking the cows, and cared for the mother and her family for some days after the birth, until she was fit to take up again the heavy work that was an integral part of life on a pioneer farm.*

These women often travelled some distance between their own homes, where they had work of their own to do, and the new mother's home. And, if a woman went into labour when the helper was in the middle of a major domestic project, the helper brought her own work along:

> *I recall one time a man coming 18 miles in a sleigh to take my grandmother to his wife who was expecting a baby. My grandmother had mixed bread dough earlier in the day, so she packed the pan of dough in with her in this sleigh, which was comfortably warm with lots of blankets and quilts and heated stones. When she arrived at the farmer's home, the dough had risen enough to bake, so she baked it in the stove in his kitchen and, after she delivered the baby, the husband drove my grandmother back home with all her bread baked.*

There was rarely any exchange of money for this kind of "turn-about" help. Families repaid each other with gifts of produce, assistance with farm work, or with building and equipping a house. The strong links forged between women at times of great significance in their lives formed a basis for the new communities that were being created.

Postnatal support was given as a matter of course too, and women sent over cooked meals for the new mother and her family. As one midwife in an isolated fishing community in Newfoundland put it, "There was always other women from around coming and looking out to things that needed to be done. No one starved, let me tell you, when a woman was lyin' in."* In this community it was the custom on the last day of lying in to have an "up-sitting day", when the neighbouring women, together with the midwife, gathered in the new mother's house for tea and "Groaning Cake", often baked by the father.*

In the past no woman had to labour alone or among strangers, and no mother lacked postnatal nurture. Isolation and loneliness came with the move from home to hospital. Even in hospital, having another woman there who is responsible to you, not to the hospital, and who has no medical function, may bring a great deal of comfort, ease labour, and result in a better outcome. When research was done in Guatemala comparing the labours of women going into hospital with no support from other women with those of others who had one-to-one support from a caring woman, even one they did not know before, the results were spectacularly in favour of the woman-to-woman support.* A Canadian study found that those women who had their partners with them and had also been assigned a "monitrice" were admitted to hospital later in labour, were more likely to require no medication during childbirth, and to have an intact perineum.*

With home birth the presence of other women in the family and female friends occurs quite spontaneously without the need to obtain permission or worry about protocol. In such a setting women rediscover an ancient role in childbirth and the postpartum weeks, and can form a strong, loving group to nurture the mother and be in company with her through a significant life transition.

"It mattered to me that the women there had had babies themselves and knew what it was like. They weren't shocked or surprised by anything. They stayed calm, down-to-earth, and always comforting."

Doctors often find the presence of other women during a birth very threatening to their professional status. Hospital nurses and midwives may feel uneasy in the same way. They fear that they will lose control of the patient. So in a hospital you may be told that there is "no room", or that they might "get in the way" or distract you and make the labour go badly.

GIVING THE RIGHT KIND OF HELP

It is undoubtedly true that a lively party going on around you during labour may prove irritating, and contradictory advice or general chat can be as intrusive, in its own way, as obstetric intervention. Any women who are with you should be able to tune in to how you are feeling and what you want of them. Michel Odent believes that the presence of other people, even the husband, may prevent a woman from trusting her instincts and from "being on another planet", as he calls the state of focused inward concentration when labour is at its height.

But when women are bonded together in a task – whether in a workplace outside the home, a kitchen, or a birth room – there is a special quality about the work they do. There is a common give-and-take in their interaction, an understanding that develops between them – often with no need for words – that can be described only by the word "sisterhood". I am not claiming that something similar cannot exist for men too – only that childbirth is a female task, and that women sharing in the spirit of birthing create an atmosphere that can give huge strength and confidence to the labouring woman.

There should be no talking during contractions, no bustling about or busyness, only a turning towards the woman in labour. She should be at the centre of everything that is happening, and her needs and wishes are paramount. If she wants to be alone, her helpers leave and wait near by. If she wants only one other person with her after all, that is her choice. There must be no conflict, no domineering attitudes, no competition to give her most help. Those present are simply watching and waiting on life.

SUPPORTING THE MIDWIFE

It is vital that there is no friction between those present, and that there is at least one person in the group who quietly supports the midwife. This is especially the case in any country where home birth is perceived by most doctors as a dangerous gamble. The midwife may need somewhere to lie down and rest if labour is slow, may welcome food and drink and perhaps a bath. She also needs strong emotional support, and to know that her work is appreciated and that she is valued as a person.

An English midwife, Caroline Flint, has written: "To work as a midwife is stressful because, to work effectively and sensitively, the midwife gives so much of herself, and she becomes so involved with and such a part of the family with which she is involved. To enable her to be a fount of such strength, a source of so much comfort, she herself must have support and cherishing!"*

When one of my daughters was giving birth in our home, using a birth pool, the second stage was very gentle and was taking a long time. I was aware that both midwives were rather tired. I went to make a pot of tea to refresh us. The senior midwife came in and said, "Sheila, you are really

"I felt close to her. There was that wonderful 'with woman' feeling."

127

confident that Tess can do this, aren't you?" We looked each other in the eyes. "Yes, I am. I have complete confidence in her." She smiled. "That's all right then," she replied, and went back to help the unfolding of this new life with increased confidence. It culminated in the triumphant birth in water of a 4.75 kg (10½ lb) vigorous baby, whose mother had an intact perineum, and next to no bleeding. As Tess lifted him up in her arms, he looked up at her, turned to us, and then back to her, and smiled.

During those hours of labour there were two midwives, both dear friends of mine, Tess's husband Jon, myself, and my husband unobtrusively taking photographs. Tess clung to Jon physically, but with each late-first-stage contraction she sought the eyes of one midwife, while the other cradled her head in a way that made her feel utterly safe. At times one of us passed her a small sponge on which to suck, brushed her hair back from her face, or gave her iced water to sip. Sometimes I held her head and the midwife and Jon held her legs. Then Jon and I held her legs and the midwife her head. And when she was out of the water she often squatted or knelt, with the midwife and her husband on either side with their arms around her and the other midwife face to face with her, giving her understanding and love.

Afterwards the senior midwife told me that when she worked on the delivery suite in the hospital in the days following she felt very alone, even though midwives there are supposed to work as members of teams. Even in a large institution where people are milling about, and perhaps especially in a large institution, a midwife can feel unsupported. The support that other women can give a midwife in an out-of-hospital birth is precious.

CHILDREN

Many women who already have children choose an out-of-hospital birth so that the older siblings can to some extent share in the birth experience, meet the new baby in an atmosphere that is warmer and more welcoming than that of a hospital, and do not have to be separated from their mother because of her admission to hospital. Yet there is more to it even than that.

All of us who approach childbirth with no experience of it, no idea of what happens except what can be gained from books and films, are in some sense deprived. Girls growing up without any awareness of what it feels like to give birth, other than the fear of pain and injury, are especially deprived. In medicalizing childbirth and removing it from the home, in separating it from the family, our culture has made birth, like dying, a fearful ordeal that can be dealt with only by trained experts, that is no longer part of our shared lives, and is out of women's control. In bringing birth back into a

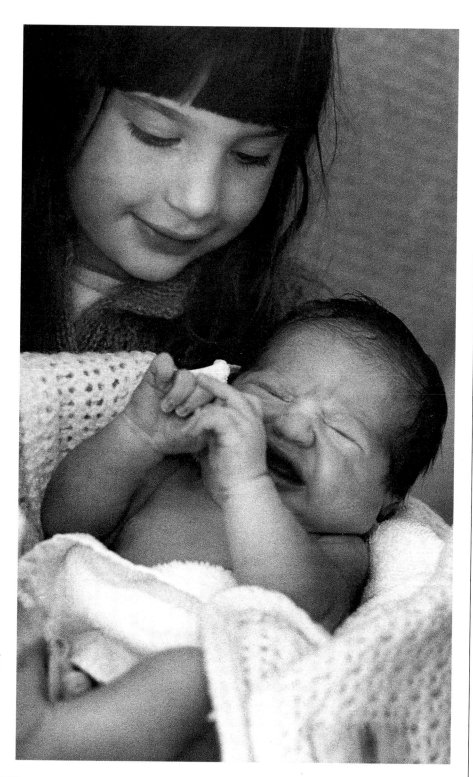

Holding in her arms a new-born who is still crumpled, warm and wet from the womb helps an older child really feel that this is "our" baby.

setting that is controlled by women, making it a family occasion, and involving the children, we reclaim it, and prepare children to reclaim it for themselves later in their own lives.

This does not mean that you sit a two-year-old down in front of you in labour and expect him to watch quietly for hours on end, or even for ten minutes, if what he really wants is to stampede around the garden in a boisterous game, or to go and feed the ducks. It does mean that he is free to go in and out to you as he wishes, can cuddle up beside you when he wants the comfort of your presence or is sleepy, can help by offering you ice chips if your mouth is dry, or a damp cloth for your forehead to cool you down. It also means that if he happens to be around when you are pushing the baby out, he is able to see what is happening, to share in the excitement of birth, and to touch and hold the new baby immediately afterwards. It will be an unforgettable experience.

"My three-year-old son saw his brother being born. When he saw the baby coming, he sang, 'Happy birthday to you'."

Women are often adamant that they would not want their older children present because it would be distracting and they would get in the way. They would have to be mothering when they wanted to concentrate on themselves. This is one effect of the isolation of women from each other and the erosion of the extended family. There is often no one else who understands what a small child wants or who can comfort him.

Having a child around when you are in labour works only if one of your helpers, someone close to you and whom he loves, has special responsibility for the child. Otherwise your birth partner will be constantly distracted from attending to your needs with changing a nappy, fetching a potty, finding the teddy bear, or kissing a hurt better. So plan ahead for this well before the time of birth, and let the child share in your plans.

"There she was, wriggling and screaming! Chris lifted her into my arms. I realized my other three kids had missed her birth. Then there they were, in the room. Each of their faces, at that moment, is fixed in my mind for ever."

Preparing your child

To prepare your child for the birth of a new baby, you may want to:

☐ Tell her how she grew and developed inside your body, using the book I have written for children, and looking together at the photographs in it of fetal development.*

☐ Make a picture book together about when your older child was a baby, and tell the story of that birth in simple language.

☐ Look at photographs of new babies and talk about their appearance, how they behave, and what they can do.

☐ If you are lucky enough to be able to do so, watch an animal birth, or see a film of animals being born.

"I agreed to look after Stephen (aged three) and take him out if he became bored. We went off and made gingerbread men in the kitchen, and then David called us back in because the baby was about to be born. She was pushing and we could soon see the crown of the baby's head. I explained what we were seeing and what was happening. With the next push the baby's head emerged. Stephen was enthralled! Soon after the baby was born, he sat in the armchair and cuddled her."

☐ Describe what happens during human birth, and how the baby's head looks when it first appears. Help the child understand the appearance and function of the umbilical cord and the placenta, and distinguish clearly between birth blood and the blood of injury.

☐ Look together at birth photographs and talk about them.

☐ Have your child meet and, if possible, hold a new baby, and watch the mother breastfeeding. Talk together about how a new baby needs to be cared for and why.

As you are doing this, remember that it is easy to overload a small child with information about birth and babies. This child wants to be the centre of your attention, and not feel rejected in favour of the new baby. So you will also want to talk about feelings: feeling alone, feeling loved, feeling excited, and feeling sad.

It is essential that your midwife knows your child too, so that she feels comfortable with the child's presence, and that the child knows her as a friend whose arrival is welcomed. They should have developed a relationship during the antenatal visits, when she explained what she was doing and why, in simple language, and got him to "help". Your older child will have already listened to the baby's heartbeats like galloping hooves, felt the baby kick, seen you practise the different positions and movements you may want to use in labour, and watched you relaxing and breathing. It is a good idea to rehearse the noises you may want to make too, so that the child is not surprised by them: grunting, moaning, panting, sighing, and groaning. Children usually take all this in their stride if they are well prepared and if they feel secure.

A child at a home birth, or one in any woman-centred setting, is witness to the care and love that is given to the mother. This is an important learning experience about human compassion, sensitivity, and tenderness. The child is witness also to the power in women, the energy in the mother, and the strength of women to help and support each other. And, if it turns out that way, the child is present as the miracle of life unfolds, hears the first cry, and sees warm, damp, crumpled flesh become a little person who can be held in her own arms and stroked.

"Olivia is seven and begged not to be left out of it. She was sitting beside me when the baby's head was born, and leant over and kissed it and said, 'Hello, baby!' I felt a wave of warmth and love for her and for everybody, and at the next push the baby slithered out. She was so excited! We all kissed and cuddled and cried with joy."

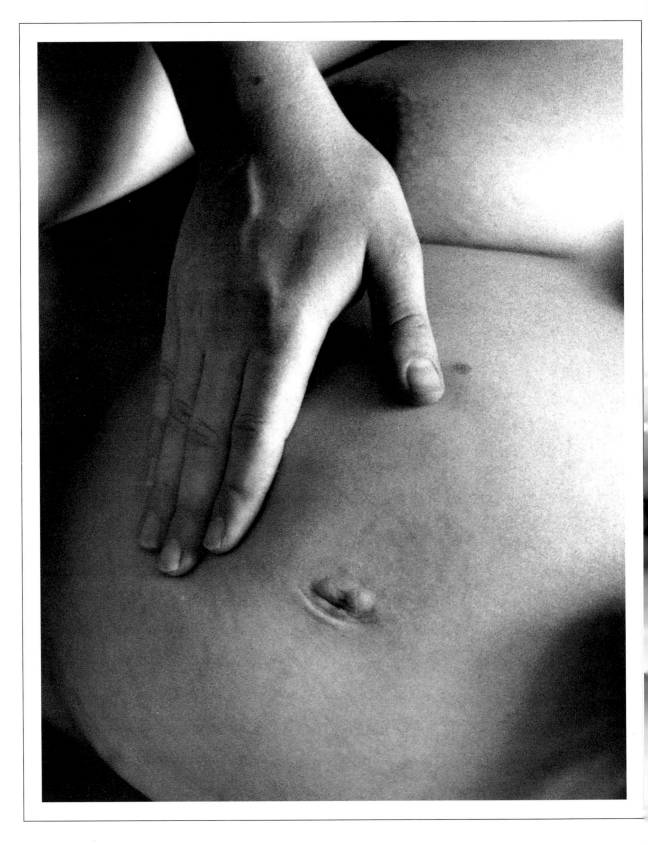

9

Meeting Challenges

All that is needed for the majority of labours to go well is a healthy, pregnant woman who has loving support in labour, self-confidence, and attendants with infinite patience. Sadly most women don't have these things, and then even a straightforward labour can become difficult, with rescue manoeuvres taking the place of the nurturing that is the basis of good midwifery care.

Women who have their babies in hospital are more likely to have difficult labours just because they are in hospital. The physiology of birth has been disturbed. They are also at risk, by virtue of being in hospital, of suffering the effects of iatrogenic medical care – that is, being subjected to interventions that themselves introduce pathology. This is not to say that problems never develop in planned out-of-hospital births, only that they are usually of a kind that can be solved by simple, non-invasive measures.

In this chapter I shall look at some of the things that can be done to help when difficulties are encountered, so that you and your midwife or doctor can discuss together what action to take.

YOU ARE OVERDUE

Most babies are not born on the date they are expected. Generally speaking, it is safer for them to be born after the expected date of delivery than preterm. Although with prolonged pregnancy every hour may seem like a week, and each week a month, a baby will usually be born within ten days of the expected date. If you go past ten days, it may be because you had a long menstrual cycle, ovulated later than you thought, and so conceived later, or because the date based on ultrasound that you were given was incorrect. Gestational age based on the known first day of the last menstruation is sometimes more accurate than ultrasound.* There is a random error of two weeks with ultrasound.*

Going for bumpy car rides or drinking gin does not start labour. Uncomfortable journeys just leave you tired and aching. Alcohol inhibits labour. Alcohol used to be given to stop preterm labour because it prevents secretion by the pituitary gland of oxytocin, the natural substance that initiates labour, and blocks the effect of oxytocin on the uterus. It may cause respiratory depression in the newborn.*

Sexual arousal

You may find that contractions start after sexual stimulation, which leads to the release of oxytocin in the bloodstream. This may have an effect similar to that of synthetic oxytocin administered through an intravenous drip in order to start labour artificially. Even what is for many women the very gentle arousal produced by nipple stimulation, carried out either by yourself or someone else, may produce contractions if continued for 20 minutes or so at a time.* It can be done by just stroking the nipples with your fingers, rolling, sucking or licking them, or by resting a warm face cloth on your breasts, lifting it off when it cools, dipping it in hot water, and pressing it against the nipples again.

With nipple stimulation contractions may at first be very short, and only gradually become longer, although in some women long, strong contractions are stimulated immediately. If they last for one minute or longer, reduce or stop the stimulation, since you may be particularly sensitive to it.

As you stimulate one nipple, you will notice that both nipples react, and may be aware of sensations in the other breast too. The same happens when you breastfeed. When the baby sucks at one breast, the milk ejection reflex occurs in both.

There is an extraordinary link between the nipples and the uterus, as you discover when you breastfeed. In the days after birth, when the baby latches

"Kathryn was originally due on 12 September, but she was born on 20 October. I was allowed to go for so long overdue as it was decided that I had not conceived until four weeks after my last period. I had only one period after coming off the Pill, and the cycle had not returned to normal."

on, you experience the warm, buzzing, milk ejection reflex as blood rushes into your breasts and, either at the same time, or soon after as the baby sucks, strong contractions of the uterus. These can be quite painful in the early days, but they are useful because they speed up your uterus's return to its pre-pregnancy size and shape.

Sexual intercourse may also stimulate contractions. This is because of the combined effect of oxytocin release and semen in the vagina. Semen is rich in prostaglandins. In fact, it is the richest source in the human body. Synthetic prostaglandins are used for induction in the form of a gel or pessary inserted in the cervix. To be most effective, semen should form a pool around the cervix. So it is back to the missionary position! Lie still for half an hour or so after your partner has ejaculated, so that the semen collects round the cervix. During this time your partner can caress your breasts so that you have both forms of stimulation.

"My doctor was muttering about induction. So we went to bed early and decided to try your method of natural induction. Contractions started, like cramps, about ten minutes after we made love, and Neil kept them going by playing with my nipples while I dozed off . . . I came to about three o'clock in the morning when contractions were coming about every five minutes. Neil was half-asleep but had one hand on the top of my tummy to feel contractions, and kept twiddling my nipple with the other. He felt very pleased with himself."

Some years ago the Japanese invented a whirring machine that could be inserted against the cervix to start contractions, because it was found that local stimulation of the tissues was effective for induction. In the absence of such a machine, and perhaps in preference to it, you might explore the effect of lying on your back with your ankles on your partner's shoulders so that his penis can be introduced deeply. This is not comfortable and should be done very, very gently. A clean finger could be used to tickle the cervix gently instead.

You can experience sexual arousal without a partner, of course. Masturbation will produce contractions and, because it is possible to have an orgasm very quickly, and to experience multiple orgasm, with self-stimulation, it may be more effective than intercourse in starting off labour.

Although breast or clitoral stimulation does not always get labour going, it may well ripen your cervix, making it soft, flexible, and thinned out, so that it dilates more easily when labour really does start.

Observing fetal movements

If you go past your due date, it may be reassuring to make a note of fetal movements. A baby who is moving vigorously is fine. Some women find fetal-movement counting worrying. Others like to be "in touch" with their babies in this way.*

Although a baby makes fewer whole-body movements in the last few weeks of pregnancy, because it is a tight fit in the uterus, a healthy baby continues to kick, often when you are resting or lying in the bath. A simple way of keeping a movement chart is to select a time of day when your baby is always at its most active and monitor what is happening during that time.

135

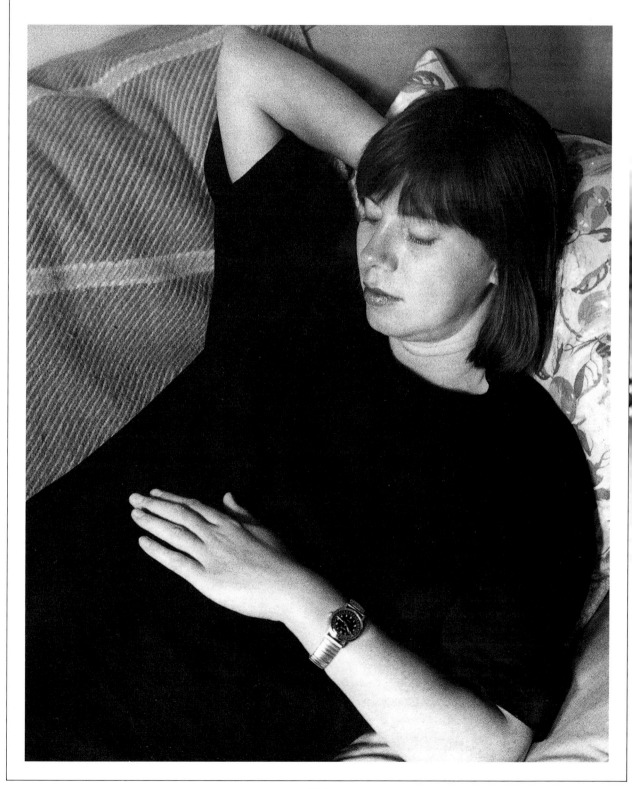

Kick chart

Take a sheet of paper and divide it up into half-hour periods like this:

Week 40	Monday	Tuesday	Wednesday	Thursday	Friday	Saturday	Sunday
3.30-4.00 p.m.							
4.00-4.30 p.m.							
4.30-5.00 p.m.							
5.00-5.30 p.m.							
5.30-6.00 p.m.							
6.00-6.30 p.m.							
6.30-7.00 p.m.							
7.00-7.30 p.m.							
7.30-8.00 p.m.							
8.00-8.30 p.m.							
8.30-9.00 p.m.							

Now count the movements up to ten, and put a tick in the square when you feel the tenth movement. An active baby continues to make its tenth movement at about the same time each day, give or take half an hour. If you find that your baby has quietened down, the most likely possibility is that labour is about to start and, in this case, there may be other signs, such as: a rush of energy as you feel the "nesting" instinct and want to clean out cupboards or finish a work project; the need to empty your bladder frequently; slight looseness of the bowels – like a minor digestive upset; low backache; a feeling that your baby's head is hanging between your legs like a coconut; and more frequent Braxton Hicks (practice) contractions of your uterus. When movements are much reduced and labour does not start, there is a chance that a baby is no longer being nourished well by the placenta. You will want to check on this, so ring your midwife or doctor and tell them what has happened, and ask them to monitor the fetal heart.

If all is well, there is no advantage in inducing labour, even if it is only a matter of taking castor oil (the old do-it-yourself way of starting labour), simply because pregnancy is prolonged. In fact there are disadvantages in induction, since it increases the chances of a Caesarean section.*

You can enjoy these last unanticipated days of pregnancy with special activities for which otherwise you will never have time – that restaurant you meant to try, the concert you thought you wouldn't be able to go to because the baby would just be born, a day with a friend, a picnic, a trip to an art gallery or museum, a play or film that you can fit in now, or a browse round antique or craft shops. Don't just sit and wait for the first twinges

Kick charts should not be just a way of checking that a baby is vigorous, but of getting in touch with each other and enjoying "conversations".

and brood over what seems by now to be an elephant pregnancy. Soon there will be a baby in your arms.

YOU THINK LABOUR HAS STARTED BUT IT HASN'T

Many women have painful contractions that *might* be the start of labour in the last few weeks before they actually go into labour. This is "prodromal" labour, and means that changes are taking place in preparation for labour *before* dilatation starts. It is a sign that contractions are beginning to soften and thin out the cervix and push down the baby's presenting part – the part of the baby nearest your cervix, usually the head. Although tiring, this may reduce the length of time you are in labour.

You may be told that you are in "false" labour. This does not mean that you are telling lies, or that your body is not working properly. What you are feeling is real. Contractions occur especially at night that may keep you awake, and may be quite regular for several hours. The problem with prodromal labour is that a woman is likely to be in a permanently alert state, waiting for further action. This is very tiring and results in a lowering of morale even before she feels regular contractions that dilate the cervix.

If this happens to you, it is important to get sleep, perhaps with a special bed-time ritual – soaking in a bath with lavender oil, and then having a hot milk drink with honey and a teaspoon of brandy or whisky in it, or a glass of wine, and listening to soothing music as you settle down with a hot-water bottle in the small of your back or against your lower abdomen. You may also need a mild analgesic, and if it is difficult to get a long stretch of sleep at night, want to make time to sleep during the day.

YOUR WATERS BREAK BEFORE LABOUR STARTS

Ten per cent of women have premature rupture of the membranes at term (when the baby is due), and eight out of ten of these start labour spontaneously within 12 hours,* although sometimes a woman has to wait as long as 24 hours before it begins. Premature rupture is more likely when there have been vaginal examinations in the weeks preceding,* so this is a good reason for declining such examinations in the last weeks of pregnancy.

When your waters break, there may be a gush of fluid or a slow trickle. If there is only a dribble of fluid, it is probably the hind waters, the part of the bubble behind the baby's head, that are leaking, and they often reseal themselves after a while. You can ignore it. If there is a gush of fluid, note whether it is clear, or stained brown or green. If it is clear, and your baby is already engaged in your pelvis, you do not need to take special action. If it is stained, the baby has emptied its bowels of meconium, a sign that it could be under stress. You should call your midwife or doctor so that the baby's position can be checked. Often any meconium present is not fresh, which is a sign that the baby was stressed some time ago. If your baby is breech, meconium is squeezed out mechanically as the bottom is pressed down, and this is not an indication that the baby is stressed.

Premature rupture of the membranes is sometimes taken as a sign that a woman is going to have a more difficult labour. But this is not so. There is no such thing as a "dry" labour, because fresh amniotic fluid is created that keeps the baby, its cord, and the surrounding tissues moist.

An important thing to know when membranes rupture is the position in which your baby is lying. So it is helpful to be aware of this at the end of pregnancy. If the baby is head down and the head is low in the pelvis, there is no possibility of the type of emergency occurring when a loop of cord slips down beneath the head (see page 140). There is a remote chance of this happening if the head is still high, however, or if the baby is lying in a less usual position – breech or transverse (across the uterus). Once your membranes have ruptured, do not put anything inside your vagina or you may introduce infection. There should be no vaginal examinations out of curiosity either. The more vaginal examinations that take place, the greater the risk of infection.

If you wait anxiously for the first contraction, you will be tired out by the time your energy is really needed. So put on a sanitary pad – change it regularly – and go to bed and sleep, do some gentle work around the house or garden, play cards, chess, or Scrabble, listen to music, or watch television. Do anything except wait.

To check that there is no infection, take your temperature every three to four hours. If there is an infection, you will become slightly feverish, and you should let your caregiver know this. When you empty your bowels, be careful to wipe from front to back, away from your vagina, so that you do not introduce bacteria from your rectum. Don't starve yourself during this wait. You may not want to eat once labour starts, so avoid a long fast now. Have plenty of fluids – fruit juice, tea, or whatever you fancy – to help replace your amniotic fluid, and keep your energy up with snacks of high-carbohydrate food, such as pasta, baked potato, and pancakes with syrup. Some midwives suggest taking supplementary vitamin C to build resistance to infection, 250 mg every few hours.*

PROLAPSED CORD

A prolapsed cord is an obstetric emergency. It occurs rarely – in 0.3 per cent of pregnancies. It happens occasionally in late pregnancy, when membranes rupture prematurely, whether or not a woman intends to have her baby in hospital. Prolapse is dangerous because the baby's oxygen supply depends on blood flowing freely through the cord. When it prolapses, the cord gets nipped between the mother's pelvis and the baby's presenting part (head or bottom). A Caesarean section is often the only way to deliver the baby safely.

Your midwife will diagnose that the baby's cord is trapped if it can be felt pulsating in your vagina, but sometimes it is too high to feel, and the clue is a marked deceleration in the fetal heart immediately following membrane rupture when the presenting part was high. **Go to hospital immediately**.

Emergency treatment of cord prolapse is to get into a knee–chest position with your bottom high in the air. Your midwife, or your birth partner if no professional caregiver is present, inserts two clean fingers in your cervix to press the baby's presenting part up and away from the cord. If you go to hospital in a car or ambulance, keep in this position with a blanket thrown over you, your pelvis raised high on a beanbag or pile of pillows, and your helper's fingers maintaining pressure inside your cervix to lift the presenting part away from it. A prolapsed cord is very unlikely to occur during a home birth or in any birthplace where invasive procedures are not practised. It is usually a consequence of intervention, in particular of rupturing the membranes artificially when the presenting part is very high.

A LONG, SLOW LABOUR

"Ross and I decided to take the dog for a vigorous walk in the park to see if we could hurry things along. It was a real pleasure, interrupted by strong contractions that began coming every ten minutes again. I sat down, or leaned against him or a tree, and he supported me through the breathing. I felt strong and confident."

It is difficult to time the onset of labour precisely and, although some women are suddenly aware that this is IT, far more experience a gentle lead-in to labour. You may decide you are in labour with contractions that are spaced about ten minutes from the start of one to the start of the next, or may adopt a "wait and see" attitude. Anxiety makes a woman more sensitive to the pre-labour phase and alerts her to action before she can do anything to help herself. It is better to relax and let things happen. Your body will tell you that you are in labour when it really needs your concentrated attention.

The shortest labours are not necessarily the best. A rapid labour can be shocking for the mother and prove stressful for the baby. In statistical terms the best outcomes follow a labour of between 12 and 24 hours for women having their first babies, and a labour lasting between 3 and 24 hours for women having subsequent babies.*

The arbitrary decision made by some obstetricians that labour must not last longer than 12 hours, or that dilatation must proceed by 1 cm per hour, puts the woman under stress and makes her attendants anxious too, so that they sometimes act unwisely in an attempt to hurry labour along. They may rupture the membranes in order to hasten a slow labour. But if this is done before 4 cm dilatation of the cervix, it can actually slow down an already slow labour. If you are already around 9 cm dilated, however, the point at which membranes usually rupture naturally, amniotomy may speed up the late first stage.*

In hospital a long, slow labour is often termed "failure to progress" only because caregivers find the waiting intolerable. Most long labours are simply variations on a theme, and there is an art in adapting to them and not being hassled or discouraged.

"If someone doesn't cover that clock, I'm going to break it!"
Woman having a hospital birth

If your labour is slow:

☐ Intersperse activity and rest, and change your activities frequently. Avoid boredom. Bake a cake for the celebration afterwards, soak in a bath, go for a walk, sew or knit – anything rather than lying in bed wondering if there is something wrong because labour is not going faster.

☐ Eat easily digested, smooth foods, such as potato purée, soup, mashed banana, ice-cream, sorbet, honey sandwiches, or yogurt, and drink plenty of fluids. In most cultures special foods are used to keep up a woman's strength in labour. In Pakistan it may be a paste of dates and sesame seeds; in China chicken ginger soup; among native women in Colombia fig juice; and in the Caribbean spice tea which, like the raspberry leaf tea popular in Europe, has a mild oxytocic action.

"We spent much of the first stage in the garden, putting in bedding plants together. Then we came in and made some biscuits and cleared up the kitchen. By that time I could tell from her breathing that she was nearly fully dilated."
A midwife talking about a client's labour

☐ Move around and keep changing position in order to stimulate uterine activity, and to encourage the baby to descend and rotate with the crown of the head against your cervix. Rock your pelvis, go up and down stairs, and lunge against the wall.

☐ Soak in a bath or have a shower to refresh you and help you to relax.

☐ Empty your bladder every hour and a half to two hours. (Your partner can keep a note of it and remind you.)

☐ A woman in slow labour welcomes quiet, calm reassurance from the attendants: "You are doing well. The baby is fine. It doesn't matter that labour is slow." You should not feel under any pressure of time. It is often good to be left alone with your birth partner.

☐ Explore what happens when you do nipple stimulation or gentle clitoral massage. You can do it yourself or ask your partner to do it. Or you could both simply get into bed, send everyone away, turn off the light, and have a cuddle for an hour.

START–STOP LABOUR

"Contractions stopped completely. I was so disappointed. I felt ready to cry. So I did cry, long and hard. Colin and I barbecued the biggest steak we could find and ate lots of salad and vegetables and potatoes to keep it company. I put an apple-sauce cake in the oven and got ready for bed. Then I felt a strong contraction and, after that, another one . . . ."

Some labours are slow in a different way. They start and then seem to stop. The uterus contracts weakly or ceases to contract for an interval, then starts again, but may have another phase of inactivity. There may be plateaux like this when nothing much seems to be happening.

A start–stop labour occurs most commonly when a woman is admitted to hospital and her previous regular, strong contractions become spasmodic and weak. The cause is anxiety. The uterus is very responsive to anxiety and this is as true for other mammals as for women. Interference can make any animal's labour more difficult. For example, when mice are disturbed during labour, their labours are prolonged and they are more likely to deliver dead pups.*

If you have a start–stop labour, try to find the cause of the anxiety. Bring it out into the open, and ask your birth partner and midwife to help you deal with it. Before you can melt into your labour, you are going to have to discard all these fears.

In many traditional cultures it is a recognized task of the midwife to help a mother in this way. She is sometimes more like a priest at confessional, listening while a woman unloads feelings of guilt and fear. She also oversees the harmonizing of relationships between the woman and those closest to her. In Greece, for example, if there has been hostility between the mother and any other woman in the village, it is believed that labour may be made difficult. The cure for this is for the other woman to come begging forgiveness and bringing water for the mother, which she drinks from the other woman's hands.

"I lay down for a couple of hours, and my contractions spaced out more. Then I got up again and found that, with walking, the intensity increased and they came every three or four minutes, lasting 45 to 60 seconds."

Keep as active as you can, unless you are very tired, in which case you could rest in a darkened room, perhaps with soft music to screen you from any disturbing sounds. Your midwife can rest near you, and many midwives bring some sewing or other work to do ready for just such eventualities.

There is a physical cause for some start–stop labours. The baby's head is in an awkward position and becomes stuck. Your midwife will monitor the fetal heart regularly and assess the situation. When a baby is awkwardly positioned, moving about and rocking and rolling your pelvis may coax the baby into a better position so that labour can progress. And even when the head is a tight fit, and the baby's descent through the pelvis is delayed, the spontaneous movements a woman makes can assist the uterus to ease the baby's head through the cervix and down the birth canal.

The diagnosis of cephalo-pelvic disproportion (CPD) is made far too often, when what is really meant is, "We couldn't be bothered to wait," or "We were afraid," or "The mother's morale dropped." If after discussion and exploring all the alternative ways of stimulating labour you decide that further action is called for, you will need to go to hospital. An oxytocin intravenous drip (syntocinon) cannot be set up at home because it is a powerful and potentially dangerous drug. For some labours it is the most effective solution to reduced uterine activity. This is not an emergency, however, and you will have time to discuss it fully and come to a decision with your midwife or doctor.

A LULL AT THE END OF THE FIRST STAGE

"Everything got very quiet, with gentle contractions like ripples. I felt drowsy and dreamy. Nothing seemed to be happening. I wondered if I'd know when to push. But there was no doubt about it. After about half an hour I suddenly felt this great wave of longing and incredible rush of energy and I shouted, 'Got to push!'."

When the baby's head is high and still above the level of the ischial spines – the bony protruberances in the pelvic cavity – there is often a pause at the very end of the first stage of labour. The uterus rests, and everyone else can rest too. In hospital, during this pause, the decision is often made to set up a syntocinon drip in order to stimulate the uterus into action.

Both in hospital and at home it is wiser to *wait* for descent and rotation of the head to occur, and at the same time give your body a chance to prepare for the active second stage. You can use this "rest and be thankful" phase to good advantage – perhaps have a shower – and come out of it refreshed and with renewed energy.

Squatting is a good position for initiating contractions and encouraging rotation of the baby's head so that it can press against your pelvic floor muscles. When the head touches nerves in these muscles, the pushing reflex is stimulated, and oxytocin spurts into your bloodstream, causing strong contractions. If you start pushing simply because you are fully dilated and have been told to do so, but do not feel the spontaneous reflex, you may become exhausted with straining, and are likely to push the baby's head down unrotated, with resulting deep transverse arrest, when the baby cannot turn its head to the easiest position for delivery. In most labours this is completely avoidable if a woman is not urged to push too soon and if everyone waits patiently.

LOW BACKACHE

One of the most difficult things to handle in labour is low backache. It continues as a gnawing ache between contractions, as well as being a sharp sacro-lumbar pain during them, and can wear down any woman's spirits. Backache occurs particularly when the baby's back is against the mother's spine (posterior position), and the hard back of the baby's extended head (that is, when the chin is lifted) is pressing against her sacrum and sacro-lumbar ligaments. Any position in which the baby can be tipped forwards on to the mother's abdominal wall and away from her spine may ease it: a forward-kneeling or all-fours position, for example, together with swinging, rocking, and circling of the pelvis. Tipping the baby forwards also helps it to rotate from the posterior to the anterior position, since it is easier for the baby to tuck its head in and turn against the abdominal muscles, especially if they are relaxed, than against the bony spine.

Firm massage or counter-pressure over the painful area is also helpful. Hot or cold compresses relieve pain too. Either a hot-water bottle or a small packet of frozen peas may work well. A strong jet of hot or cold water directed on to the spot as pain builds up often brings blessed relief. Some women labouring in water find that massage while they are in a forward-leaning position in the birth pool or bath provides amazing pain-relief.

Transcutaneous electronic nerve stimulation (TENS) helps some women, but proves irritating or ineffective for others. TENS is done by means of a hand-held instrument, about the size of a small camera, which sends electrical impulses to the brain to block pain messages. It is battery-operated, with four electrodes which are attached with adhesive tape at either side of the spine, two with their upper edges at the level of the lower ribs and two in the lower back. The woman controls its operation herself and can move about, lie down, or sit up. It seems to be less effective for abdominal than for back pain.

The instrument's low-frequency current produces a buzzing sensation, which is thought to stimulate the release of endogenous (internal) opiates and endorphins into the cerebro-spinal fluid, thus raising tolerance of pain and increasing the sense of wellbeing.* If you know before the onset of labour that your baby is posterior, it can be worth hiring, borrowing, or buying TENS equipment. It may reduce backache, and, even when it does not, enables you to feel more positive about your labour, because it is something you can do to help yourself, and is harmless to the baby.*

Any woman with severe backache needs her helpers' undivided attention, and generous encouragement to keep going. Because pain of this kind is very wearing, she may feel unable to continue to move about. If this happens to you, flop forwards, spreadeagled over a beanbag, so that your partner can reach your back and massage or press against it. The position will help the baby's head to rotate. Or lie on your side in what the French obstetrician Pierre Vellay calls the "jack-knife position". This is simply three-quarters-over side-lying (the recovery position) with your underneath arm spread out behind you, all your limbs well flexed, and your head bent forwards. You will spontaneously select the correct – because more comfortable – side on which to lie. Most posterior babies lie with the back on the mother's right: the right occipito posterior (ROP) position. This is five times more common than left occipito posterior (LOP). If your baby is ROP, lie on your left side with your top knee drawn up and pressing against your abdomen. This encourages the baby to tip forwards into a position where it is easier for it to turn to the anterior. If your baby is LOP, you will be more comfortable on your right side, and this helps the baby turn.

If you choose this position, your birth partner can sit close against your lower back, with the side of his pelvis pressing hard against the area where you feel most pain. You will find the right spot after a little experiment. Then you can have the whole weight of his body leaning against you at the peak of pain. He can also massage your back by rocking his own pelvis.

Once the baby rotates, backache may vanish almost miraculously, and you go straight into the pushing stage. When I was doing anthropological field work in Jamaica, I found that the shape of many women's pelvises was such that their babies were posterior for a long time in labour. They disliked the backache but welcomed it as a sign that the "gate" in their backs was creaking open to let the baby out. If you think of that pain as a gate opening, it may be easier to bear. Once it is open wide, you know that the baby is almost with you.

MORALE DROPS

Most women feel that they can't go on and would like to postpone having the baby when they reach the end of the first stage of labour. These feelings are a sign of progress: for this is transition, the bridge between the first and second stage. You long for some rest from the storm of contractions and may get very irritable. In a long labour, or one with backache, you are likely to feel discouraged earlier than this, and it is up to those helping you to give you strong, cheerful, concentrated emotional support.

The words that are used, and the tone in which they are said, are of first importance. There is no formula that is right for every woman. But a good

"It was painful. My midwives told me that they knew it was hard for me but that the baby was fine. That made all the difference."

"The three hours that transition lasted seemed endless. 'When will this be over?' I kept muttering. The pain no longer seemed localized low in my abdomen. It overtook my whole body. It was huge and overwhelming."

midwife has phrases that express her nurturing personality, her conviction that the woman can do it, in a way that is sympathetic and empowering for the woman.

Some midwives have written about this in detail, and I can almost hear my friend Caroline Flint murmuring these encouraging words – similar to the ones I find myself using when I am with a woman in labour:

> *Good . . . Excellent . . . You're doing so well . . . You're beautifully relaxed . . . Let it happen . . . Let it come . . . Let it open you up . . . Surrender to it . . . Feel yourself opening up . . . Good, good, good . . . Well done . . . That's wonderful . . . That's marvellous . . . Oh, how brilliant . . . That's lovely . . . Blossom . . . Flourish . . . Open up to it . . . Be soft . . . Be giving . . . Surrender to it . . . Give, give, give . . . Surrender . . . Open, open . . . Good . . . Good, good . . .**

However tired she is, the midwife should never use these words mechanically. They express her inner awareness that the woman needs to release all tension, find her body's rhythms, and open wide.

Elizabeth Davis, midwife in San Francisco, uses such phrases as: "Keep it loose," and "Be really open and let that force move through you, just let it be, let it down."*

Penny Simkin, a childbirth educator in Seattle, has what she calls the "take charge routine" for any time in labour when a woman hits an emotional low, weeps, wants to give up, is very tense, or is in a great deal of pain. The birth partner or midwife moves in close to the mother to help her regain her inner strength. She speaks in a calm, confident voice, as she says:

> *Breathe with me . . . BREATHE WITH ME . . . That's the way . . . just like that . . . Good . . . STAY WITH IT . . . just like that . . . LOOK AT ME . . . Stay with me . . . Good for you . . . It's going away . . . Good . . . Good . . . Now just rest, that was so good.*

Between contractions she may say:

> *With the next one let me help you more. I want you to look at me the moment it starts. We will breathe together so it won't get ahead of us. Okay? Good, you're doing so well. We're really moving now.**

If there comes a time in labour when you are discouraged, you need *change*.

☐ Change your position or the kind of movements you are making.

☐ Have a change of scene. Move to another room or out-of-doors. Open the window for a while, or go to the bathroom.

☐ Try changing the rhythm of your breathing. If you were tending to breathe fast, now breathe more slowly and fully. If you were breathing deeply, let your breathing speed up and allow it to "dance" a little.

☐ Ask for a change in the kind of touch you are receiving, on a different place on your body, or a different kind of massage. Have your helpers switch over so that you are held or massaged by someone else.

☐ If other people to whom you feel close are available, ask one of them to come and be with you for a while. A fresh face often works wonders.

☐ If you have been in semi-darkness, now light a lot of candles or turn the lights up. If the room is bright, draw the curtains or dim the lights.

☐ If you have music in the background, change the tape and select a completely different rhythm and mood.

☐ Change the essential oils in your massage oil, from lavender to pine, from frankincense to juniper or orange, for example.

☐ If you have had your eyes closed during contractions, open them now, and make eye contact with your birth partner or your midwife. If you have been in eye contact until now, try closing your eyes and sinking down into yourself near the source of the power released deep in your body.

☐ Perhaps you have been silent during contractions. Now open up and make low sounds that go right down into your pelvis. Or, if you have already been making a great deal of noise, try the effect of just listening to the sound of your own breathing during contractions, and let each breath sound like a wave on the shingle.

☐ Make an opportunity to freshen up. Splash your face with cold water. Get someone to brush your hair back slowly from your face. Have a bath or shower. Suck cracked ice.

☐ Pep up your energy with a glucose drink or spoonfuls of honey eaten straight from the pot.

A woman who disciplines and trains her body, who is an athlete, swimmer, climber, dancer, or regular jogger, for instance, may lose heart if she faces difficulties in labour. She is used to mastering her body and now feels that it has let her down.

It is often claimed that dancers and horse-riders have hard labours because their pelvic floor muscles are thick. But a well-exercised muscle is also a flexible muscle. It can be contracted or released at will. The problem is more likely to be that a woman who "goes for the burn" dominates her body with stamina and courage, and can fight her labour longer. Muscular exertion will not help her in childbirth. She needs to surrender control of her muscles, and then her uterus can work for her.

Ina May Gaskin, midwife at the alternative-style community, The Farm, in Tennessee, describes how she attended a cyclist who had already been in labour for 24 hours and was becoming discouraged. She says:

> *I was pretty sure that her problem had been that, in not really "welcoming" each rush, she was actually fighting labor in a subtle but effective way.*
>
> *Then I asked her what had been the longest she had ever ridden her bicycle in one day. She looked at her husband, and together they said, 120 miles, and smiled. I said, "Having a baby is a lot like that. It takes endurance. But you have to learn a different way of pedaling." That seemed to make sense to her. I explained that she needed to be aware of the sensations that came with each rush and try to help open up and relax when each one came. I suggested that smooching would often aid the process. I left them alone for approximately 45 minutes, after which they called me back to check her dilation.*
>
> *By this time she was nearly fully dilated and was about to begin spontaneous pushing. She loved pushing and delivered her baby quite easily without a tear.**

WORRIES ABOUT THE FETAL HEART-RATE

The important thing about the baby's heart-rate is that, if it slows a lot as contractions reach their peak, it should pick up again about 15 seconds after the end of a contraction. If it does this, the baby is receiving sufficient oxygen.

The easiest way for your midwife or doctor to monitor this in an out-of-hospital labour is by using Doppler ultrasound, in the form of a sonic aid held against your abdomen over the baby's heart, to listen intermittently to the heart for a full 30 seconds following a contraction. The sonic aid can be used, whatever your position, even under water if it is first placed in a polythene bag or a condom. It leaves you free to move and, because you also hear the sound, keeps you, as well as the midwife, informed.

If the fetal heart slows down to below 100 beats per minute and does not recover in the interval between contractions, it is possible that this baby is finding it hard-going. The problem may be that the cord has been pressed between the baby and your pelvis, and this can be solved if you change position. Explore the effect of some different positions, meanwhile monitoring carefully. If you have been sitting or lying down, for instance, try standing or an all-fours position. If you are already in the second stage and have been holding your breath to push, try breathing instead, keeping your throat open. This is difficult if you are already in a pattern of breath-holding. It may help to blow out when the urge to push comes. Sometimes the baby just needs you to breathe more regularly, to keep on taking in oxygen, for it to have an easier birth. Your midwife or doctor will be carrying oxygen in case the baby needs a whiff after birth, and may have an oxygen mask for you to use at this point.

If, despite all your efforts, transfer to hospital becomes necessary, it is not failure. You have managed well up to this stage, but now need the extra help that only the hospital can provide.

Once in hospital, continuous electronic fetal monitoring may be carried out, with an electrode attached to the baby's scalp. Although this provides a continuous print-out, it is impossible to diagnose fetal distress accurately from it. One way of obtaining further information is to prick the baby's scalp and take a few drops of blood to be analysed. On the basis of the result you may be advised to have a forceps or vacuum extraction delivery or a Caesarean section. Or the doctors may think that it is "better to be safe than sorry" and decide, without further investigation, to deliver the baby immediately by one of these methods. This will be a shock for you but, after all your hard work, it may be what you want too.

YOU ARE HYPERVENTILATING

Hyperventilation is the result of breathing in and out fast and furiously. It often happens at the end of the first stage, when contractions are coming at two-minute intervals. The woman breathes too heavily, and allows no time for the slight pauses that come naturally between inspiration and expiration and between expiration and inspiration. She feels light-headed, giddy, and nauseous, has tingling fingers, is numb around the mouth, starts to sweat, and may feel terribly panicky. Physiologically she has an increased pulse-rate, a rise in blood pH (which means that the blood becomes more acidic), and blood flow to her brain decreases. A healthy baby copes well with the mother's over-breathing in labour, but a baby who is not in good condition could be harmed by this flushing out of carbon dioxide because, when this occurs, oxygen is more firmly bound to haemoglobin and cannot be easily extracted by the cells. As a result the baby gets less oxygen.*

People often hyperventilate when under stress. Labour, especially the late first stage, is stressful. It may help if, as each contraction reaches a peak, your midwife or birth partner says: "Half-way there," or "It'll soon be over now," and uses touch to give you confidence and comfort.

You can avoid hyperventilating by keeping your shoulders and throat relaxed, by focusing on the idea of relaxing a little more with each breath out, and by letting your breathing flow rhythmically. Your helpers can breathe with you so that you do not feel so alone.

If you hyperventilate, your partner can rest both hands on your shoulders and ask you to relax them and breathe more gently, with a slow sigh out. If you find this hard to do, it may help to breathe into a paper bag so that you can inhale the carbon dioxide you have exhaled. As you do this, focus on the short pause after each breath in and each breath out.

YOU BECOME VERY TIRED

Labour is an intense, energy-consuming activity, and may be the most strenuous work you have ever done. A woman often feels as if she is on a treadmill of contractions. The suggestions listed on pages 146 and 147 will be useful now.

In many hospitals there is a rule that a woman in labour must not eat anything, because of the danger of her aspirating the contents of her stomach if she were to have a general anaesthetic. This can happen largely because gastric emptying is delayed when a woman has narcotic drugs – pethidine, for example – to relieve pain. Her only chance of being fed is through glucose and fluids received via an intravenous drip. She is bound to be exhausted if she is starving, especially if she is vomiting too. She has to draw on her fat reserves for energy, with the result that she becomes dehydrated and ketones, which are produced by metabolization of fat, appear in her urine.*

A woman having her baby in an out-of-hospital setting is unlikely to have analgesics that delay gastric emptying and is able to drink when she wishes and to eat according to her appetite. So ketosis occurs less often in birth at home. But if labour is very tiring, here are some simple remedies:

☐ Have a drink that will adjust your body's electrolyte balance. One that has been devised by American home birth midwives is called "Labor-Aid".*

You can make it by mixing together 1 quart water, ⅓ cup honey, ⅓ cup lemon juice, ½ teaspoon salt, ¼ teaspoon baking powder, and 2 crushed calcium tablets.

☐ Eat something that does not need much chewing and can just slip down. You may fancy a pot of frozen yogurt or fromage frais, some smooth porridge with honey or syrup, or a few spoonfuls of mashed mango. These will give you instant energy.

☐ Do not fight the pain. Go right into it instead. Resisting it means that you are not allowing your body to open up. A surprising release can come when we accept pain and go with it.

☐ Whatever happens during contractions, ensure that you are resting completely in each interval between. Drop forwards on to pillows placed conveniently. It is often possible to sleep for half a minute before the next contraction starts. Ask your birth partner to rest a hand on your abdomen and tell you softly when the next one is starting, so that you can tune in to it and not be taken by surprise.

☐ Remember that you are having a baby. It is easy to forget this when you are in the thick of labour. One midwife friend of mine often borrows a baby to bring to the woman in labour when she is at this stage, just to remind her of what it is all about. A birth partner or a midwife says: "Come on, baby! Come on down. Come on, baby – just a little more." This may give you fresh heart.

"After five hours I was beginning to tire of riding the pains. Anne was encouraging me all the time, saying: 'Relax into it – you're doing very well – very good.' She put a sponge in my mouth and I sucked on it, and she wiped my face with a warm, damp flannel. She said to me: 'Don't worry about other people. Just breathe. Keep breathing. You are doing it. You've made it. Well done!' The midwife said I was only 5-6 cm dilated. Anne said, 'You know it goes much more quickly from now on.'"

YOU HAVE A PUSHING URGE BEFORE BEING FULLY DILATED

A woman may have the desire to push before her cervix is fully open. Pushing hard against an incompletely dilated cervix can make it puffy and swollen so that it actually closes a little. This must make labour more difficult for the baby. If you want to push and are not yet 10 cm dilated, you may find the following suggestions helpful:

☐ Continue breathing. Do not hold your breath. When the longing to push comes, give two quick breaths out followed by one slow breath out, so that there is a steady rhythm of pant, pant, blow, breathe in. It sometimes helps if your birth partner holds up a finger in front of your mouth, so that you can direct each blow on to it. As soon as the urge leaves you, breathe fully and easily again.

☐ If you are in an upright position, this is the time to change it and lie down on your side or be on all fours. This will have the effect of slightly reducing the pressure of the baby's head against your rectum and anus, so that you don't feel so desperate to push.

☐ If you *have* to push, do so with an open mouth and breathing *out*. Let your uterus do the work while you open up.

YOU GET NO PUSHING URGE

A woman can have a baby without *deliberately* pushing it out. Her uterus sees to that. The energy that she gives to expulsion is only a small part – 30–40 per cent – of the power that is exerted by her uterus to press the baby down through the cervix, the folds of her vagina, and the spreading tissues of her perineum.

Until there is an irresistible urge to push, it is sensible to avoid pushing by continuing to breathe. There is no need to hold your breath at all. In this way, all the tissues have a chance to fan out smoothly before the ball of the baby's head eases through, with no damage to ligaments, muscles, or skin.

Many women and birth attendants hope to hurry the birth along by pushing before the mother's body is quite ready. This can only do harm and is very tiring. Once the baby's head touches nerves in her perineum, the Ferguson reflex is stimulated, endogenous oxytocin is released, and she feels the impulse to push.*

For some women this does not happen until the baby is just about to be born. The mother pushes once or twice and the baby slips out easily.

Sometimes the desire to push is there, but is not strong. That's fine too. Go with your body. "Listen" to your uterus. When the second stage has started passionately, some gentler contractions may follow in which the pushing urge is faint or non-existent. For a woman who is really free to follow her uterus, the pushing rhythm which it dictates may vary with different contractions. Some pushes are short and others long. Sometimes there is only one push with a contraction, at other times four or five. Even if you feel unsure about what to do, your body *knows* how to give birth.

MECONIUM IS PASSED

The bowels of a mature fetus contain meconium, and if the baby is under stress this meconium is expelled in the amniotic fluid. The presence of meconium is a sign of maturity, but it can also mean that the baby is stressed. If the baby inhales meconium, there is a chance that respiratory-tract infection can develop.

Meconium is brown and sticky when fresh, green when stale. The passage of stale meconium is a sign that the baby may have been stressed in the past. If the baby is about to be born and fresh meconium is passed, your midwife or doctor will simply have a mucus extractor ready to suck out meconium gently – even before the baby's body is born, and before the chest has expanded to take the first breath.

It will be easier to do this if you stand with your knees bent or are on all fours, with your midwife or doctor behind you. Breathe the baby out gently, rather than pushing, and there will be time for your caregiver to suction out every bit of meconium.*

If you are nowhere near birth when meconium is passed, your attendants will probably suggest that you transfer to hospital so that a paediatrician can be ready to resuscitate a "flat" baby and make sure that the airways are clear by suctioning out any contents, using an endotracheal tube if necessary. "Flat" does not refer to a baby's shape, but to vitality at birth. A "flat" baby is limp and floppy, and breathing is depressed.

You may feel frightened about the need for transfer. Most babies who have passed meconium during labour are perfectly all right, but having a paediatric check-up and making sure that the baby's respiratory tract is clear means that you take no chances.

THE BABY IS COMING VERY FAST

"Sometimes, while helping a mother through crowning, I feel like I'm outside a semi-trailer truck, directing the driver: 'All right, bring it on a little now – hold it for a few seconds now. Okay, bring it on some more.' While she holds back that tremendous force, the whole quality of her skin will change – she will relax and become more pliant and stretchy."
A midwife*

When the second stage is rapid – known as a precipitate second stage – and it looks as if the baby will pop out like a champagne cork, there are several things you can do to slow down the pace and make the birth gentler:

☐ Adopt an all-fours position, or lie on your side, so that your midwife or doctor can "guard" your perineum with a hand. Do not squat or stand.

☐ Breathe the baby out. Guide your baby down with your breathing. Avoid pushing. If you have to push, breathe again as soon as possible.

☐ Release your pelvic floor muscles and relax your perineum, by opening your mouth, dropping your jaw, and opening your glottis. Imagine a ripe fruit with all its seeds spilling out, or even a tube of toothpaste that you have accidentally stood on, with the toothpaste oozing out, or perhaps a waterfall with a great rush of water pouring through the rocks – whatever image best helps you relax.

☐ If you want to make noises, moo, bellow, groan, or give deep sighs – resonant sounds that go right down into your pelvis. Do not scream or yelp. That will make you tighten up.

☐ Listen closely and be guided by your midwife or doctor. If you are told to push, however, it is better to release tension and open up, letting your pelvic floor descend like a lift down to the basement, rather than to hold your breath and push deliberately. Then your baby can glide out, without being forcibly ejected.

If you don't want to miss the birth, remember to open your eyes and reach out your arms as soon as you feel the baby slither from your body.

THE BABY IS A SURPRISE BREECH

Occasionally labour is going well and the birth attendants see something emerging that looks like a very bald head, and realize, perhaps after meconium is squeezed out, that it must be the baby's bottom. It is an undiagnosed breech.

Breech labour is like any other labour up to the point when the baby's body slips out. What may then happen is that the head gets stuck, which is why in hospitals when a breech is delivered vaginally – and many are delivered by Caesarean section – a large episiotomy is done and forceps are applied to the after-coming head. Actually most of any damage results from anxiety and rough handling by the person who is delivering. I have seen a doctor become anxious and pull on the baby's legs, so that the arms extended and the baby was completely stuck. A breech baby should always be delivered gently to avoid injury to the spinal cord, arms, and neck.

Left to itself, the baby's body uncurls, the uterus keeps the head flexed, and one or both legs drop out, followed by the body and then the head. In a series of 89 breech births delivered by midwives in New Jersey, USA, there was no single case of extended arms, and all the babies were fine.*

It is unwise to plan a breech delivery at home, because your baby may need help to breathe, and a paediatrician should be available. But if you have a surprise breech, adopt a supported, upright position, legs wide apart and knees bent, in order to give the baby's head most space, and to enable gravity to help it slip through. Michel Odent, the French doctor who has tried to give birth back to women, says that he would "never risk a breech delivery with the mother in a dorsal or semi-seated position".*

The worst possible position for a breech delivery is lying on your back with legs raised in lithotomy stirrups, as most hospitals recommend. In that position your sacrum and coccyx are pressed up and the dimensions of your pelvic cavity and outlet are reduced. If you squat, however, you gain an extra centimetre across your pelvic cavity and two centimetres from front to back.*

Once you have adopted a half-standing, half-squatting position, leaning on your birth partner in front of you, your midwife or doctor should be positioned behind you, and should simply wait and watch until the baby's body is completely born. The only intervention that may be necessary is to press gently behind the baby's knees if the feet are up over the shoulders. This will stimulate the baby to bend the knees so that they come down. When the legs are extended, they splint the spine, so that it is more difficult for the baby to take the curve of the birth canal.

As you bend your knees and go into a deep squat, holding on to your birth partner, the baby's body will slip out. The cord may slide down too, and if it is wrapped tightly around the baby, your midwife or doctor will carefully unloop it, but only very gently, or it may go into spasm. You may feel a confusing, intermittent pushing urge. Avoid pushing if you can until the head is ready to emerge. Let the baby be born by uterine activity alone. This will enable everything to open up and your tissues to spread wide. As soon as the whole body is born, drop forwards, legs still wide apart and knees bent, leaning over some furniture or your birth partner so that your back is almost horizontal. This tilts your pelvis so that the baby's nose and mouth are visible, and whoever is catching the baby can aspirate the nose and mouth with a mucus extractor before the head is fully born. A breech baby often begins to breathe once its chest is born, and may inhale mucus from your birth canal. The mucus can block the nasal passages, and although most babies are clever at sneezing out anything that is irritating, in this case aspiration is a wise precaution.

The decision has to be made as to whether or not to perform an episiotomy. Sometimes it is necessary in order to give the head more space.

Then you will feel the crowning, with the sensation of heat and prickling that normally precede the birth, as the widest part of the baby's head passes over your perineum.

Your midwife or doctor may wrap a warm towel around the baby's body and support the head as it slides out. A breech baby may need a few whiffs of oxygen and some massage to recover from the shock of birth.

"Then came the crowning. As quickly as this rush of contractions came, it stopped. I felt hot and high. I was excited. After climbing a very high mountain, I could now sit and enjoy the exhilarating view. I love this part of labour – the calm, high, ready feeling. My next contraction began, and I greeted it with satisfaction. Surprised by its intensity, I let my body do it."

SHOULDER DYSTOCIA

When a baby is vertex (head down), sometimes a big head is born, and then there is a delay in the delivery of the shoulders. Very rarely the shoulders really are stuck: this is known as shoulder dystocia. The midwife or doctor can see that the baby's head is large, the cheeks are fat, and the face looks squashed. There is no sign of the neck, because it is wedged inside by the broad shoulders.

Shoulder dystocia may occur because the woman has had oxytocin stimulation of the uterus which has produced artificially strong contractions that have forced the pace, propelling a big baby along the birth canal before all the tissues have fanned out. The head shoots out, and the shoulders are impacted. Women giving birth out of hospital should never have labour stimulated with oxytocin, so labour tends to be slower and gentler.

Deliberate forceful pushing with prolonged breath-holding may also eject a baby's head before the tissues have fanned out sufficiently, and because of this the shoulders are a tight fit. It seems better to allow labour to proceed at its own pace.

The head is the largest part of the baby and is like a ball that can turn on the shoulders. When the baby is nestled down, back rounded, limbs flexed, and chin tucked in, the body is like a ball too. The head can rotate and move more or less independently of the body because of the neck, and the shoulders can rotate more or less independently of the head. If big shoulders are square on, the shoulders need to rotate so that first one can slip out, then the other.

Hospital doctors employ a range of techniques to deal with shoulder dystocia. These include pressure over the woman's pubis, a large episiotomy, fundal pressure applied over the baby's bottom, the Wood "screw" manoeuvre that entails pushing the fingers inside and then pulling the baby out with a screwing motion, and the "Zavanelli manoeuvre", which involves pushing the head back in again and then delivering the baby by Caesarean section.*

If your baby's head is born and then nothing happens, *move*! Movement itself often releases the shoulders. Your birth partner should help you change position. Your midwife or doctor may ask you to get on hands and knees. The antero–posterior diameter (from front to back) of your pelvis increases by as much as one or two centimetres in this position. When the next contraction comes, push hard as your helper applies gentle downwards traction to the head. The baby sometimes falls out.*

Another very good position is to stand with your knees as wide apart as possible. Caroline Flint believes that it probably does not matter exactly how a woman moves her pelvis, "from lying down to hands and knees; from kneeling to standing up; from standing up to being on all fours – but it is important for the movement to include a tilting of the pelvis".* This pelvic tilt occurs automatically whenever you bend one knee so as to get up into a standing position, to stride forwards, or get down on the floor.

If your baby still does not budge, your helper will reach in with two fingers and find the baby's posterior armpit, the one nearest, and either pull the shoulder forwards or pull down the arm. Ina May Gaskin says that a colleague of hers safely delivered a 6.25 kg (14 lb) baby in this way. She considers that episiotomy is usually unnecessary.

TWINS

The mother of twins is more likely to develop high blood pressure and pre-eclampsia, and twins are at greater risk than singleton babies, especially the second baby. The babies are often preterm and of low birth weight. One or other may lie in a difficult position. The second baby may be high, so that a loop of cord can come down before the baby's presenting part has descended. Both babies may need intensive care for the first days or weeks of their lives.

Having said this, I had my own twins at home. I was healthy, with only mild hypertension, the pregnancy went to term, the babies were known to be a good weight and were both head down, and I had an experienced midwife and a supportive partner. These are all important factors that have to be considered.

Labour was brief: they were both born in 90 minutes, one 10 minutes after the other. If I had made the journey to hospital, they would probably have been delivered in the car. I am glad that I weighed the risks and benefits of going to hospital and made the decision to stay at home, though I remained flexible about switching to hospital if labour was not going well, or if the babies were not in good condition. I had to make the decision without my midwife. When she arrived, she advised me to go to hospital. I asked her to examine me first. She found that the head of the first baby was already on the perineum. There was then no question of moving.

If you have undiagnosed twins, or labour with diagnosed twins proceeds too quickly to risk getting to hospital:

☐ Warm the room and fill hot-water bottles so that the babies will not become cold. Small babies are quickly chilled.

☐ Stay calm and peaceful, even though this is very exciting. Breathe with a gentle expiration, as slowly as you comfortably can. You are breathing for your babies.

☐ Once in the second stage, take it as gently as possible and avoid both hyperventilating (see page 149) and prolonged breath-holding. Your first baby may cope well with these, but the second baby needs good oxygenation for a while longer.

☐ Choose any position that is comfortable for you – preferably an upright one (standing, squatting, kneeling, or half-kneeling, half-squatting). If labour is progressing very rapidly, get on all fours.

☐ When the first baby is born, put her to your breast. The sucking will stimulate further contractions to bring the next baby to birth.

A drug to stimulate uterine contractions (syntometrine) should *never* be given before the second twin is born. It results in gripping contractions of the uterus that can sometimes trap the second baby.

After the first baby is born, your midwife or doctor clamps and cuts the cord, checks the lie of the second baby and listens to the fetal heart. There is space now to adjust the baby to the best position if the lie needs correcting. If labour has not started again in 15 minutes, the usual practice is to rupture the membranes. But, if the firstborn is already suckling at your breast, this will stimulate further contractions that help the second baby towards birth, and there may then be no need to rupture the membranes artificially.

After the birth you will sweat a lot. Even though you may feel cold and shivery, you are giving out a great deal of heat, so hold both babies against you and snuggle under the bedcovers to keep them beautifully warm.

THE BABY WHO IS SLOW TO BREATHE

Babies are enormously adaptable. They can manage with very little oxygen for much longer than an adult. Some babies start to breathe as soon as their heads are born. Most take a few seconds to get going. Some start to breathe, but then breathe fitfully for as long as 20 minutes. It takes time for them to adjust. They need to be kept warm and to be touched.

When the cord is not clamped immediately, and it is pulsating, the baby is still receiving some oxygenated blood straight into her bloodstream. There need be no rush to force her to breathe.

Some babies can't breathe well because the respiratory tract is plugged with sticky mucus. When a baby is born with the mother in an upright position, any mucus drains naturally from the mouth and nose. Newborn babies often sneeze mucus out very effectively, too. If a baby needs help to breathe, the first thing to do is to make sure that the airways are clear. She can be placed on her front with the head lower than the hips, so that mucus drains out, while you, or a helper, gently massage her back.

The baby's mouth can be suctioned gently too, using a mucus extractor. It is important not to stimulate the gag reflex by putting the bulb syringe down her throat.

Babies are more likely to have breathing problems when they are born preterm and the lungs are still immature, or when they are born in a hospital where narcotic drugs, such as pethidine, have been given to the mother in high doses.

In spite of the general assumption that babies are slapped on their bottoms to encourage them to breathe, the vast majority of those who are making a slow transition do not benefit from violent stimulation of this kind. If a baby seems dopey and drugged from pain-killers in the mother's bloodstream, her feet can be tickled and, if necessary, a stimulant drug can also be injected.

A baby who has had a difficult transition to life needs warmth. Otherwise she uses up a great deal of energy trying to maintain body heat. Most heat loss is from the head, because it is the biggest part. So she should be wrapped in warmed flannel blankets and her head covered. Sometimes a baby is completely floppy and grey and needs oxygen quickly, either mouth-to-mouth or from a bag-mask. Every midwife or doctor attending a birth should carry resuscitation equipment for the rare situation in which this is needed.

In some hospitals in Eastern Europe and the USSR a baby who is slow to breathe is still put under a cold tap. In most hospitals elsewhere a baby who requires resuscitation is put on a special sloping shelf on her back, a tube is pushed down her throat, she is mechanically ventilated, and then given oxygen by face-mask. Elizabeth Davis says that she has witnessed babies whose condition worsens with this treatment, or who struggle to establish their own rhythms. "I usually find myself saying, 'Somebody touch that baby!' Or I move over and do it myself. Observation and participation has taught me that touch usually brings swift and dramatic improvement."*

There can be a spiritual element in helping a baby to life. Elizabeth Davis also writes of babies being tired after a long labour and a mother being too exhausted to welcome a baby. "You use your heart in moments like these. 'What a gorgeous girl [or boy] you have!' Or to the sibling standing by, 'You have a sister [or brother]!' There is a tangible quality of energy that kindles life and response, pure, strong, and loving, and it's the midwife's job to work with everything she's got to initiate this at the given moment."*

If a baby is just flickering and is starting, but not quite managing, to breathe, it helps to *talk* to the baby: to say "Hello, baby," "Come on love, come on!" or "You're beautiful!" The result may be that the lungs open wider, breaths are deeper, and respiration is more regular. In intensive care nurseries, where babies are being monitored very carefully, oxygen levels often rise when a baby is stroked and when the mother speaks to her baby.

YOU HAVE HEAVY BLEEDING

It is always alarming to see blood coming from your vagina during pregnancy, even if it is only a few spots. In late pregnancy you may notice slight bleeding after a vaginal examination, and sometimes after sexual intercourse. This is almost always a sign that the cervix is thin, soft, and vascular, and may have started to dilate a little already. Occasionally it is caused by a cervical polyp that has broken from its stem. This kind of bleeding stops of its own accord.

The show that often heralds labour is a blood-stained mucus plug, which can resemble the start of a period. Labour will probably begin within 24 hours after a show, although sometimes a woman goes as long as a week before contractions start. You may have several shows during labour, each heavier than the one before. This is normal.

Antepartum haemorrhage

Real bleeding is a different matter. A steady flow of blood or continual spotting can mean that the placenta is starting to peel away from the lining of the uterus (placental abruption) or that it is in front of the baby's head (placenta praevia). Let your midwife or doctor know what is happening. They will probably get you into hospital as quickly as they can, as an examination should only be done once everything has been set up for Caesarean section, should it be necessary.

Such antepartum haemorrhage may occur wherever a woman decides to have her baby, and is not a risk particularly associated with out-of-hospital birth. It is much more common in women who smoke heavily. But every woman should know the symptoms just in case it happens to her.

Bleeding in the third stage

After the baby is born your uterus continues to contract, although you may not be aware of it. The placenta cannot contract, so it peels away from the lining of the uterus, usually within half an hour of the birth, and slips down into your vagina. When this happens and the placenta is ready to be expelled, some bright-red blood appears and the cord lengthens.

The third stage of labour, the time from the birth of the baby until the delivery of the placenta, can be conducted in two ways:

☐ Active management entails an injection of syntometrine – usually into the mother's thigh – as the baby is born, early cord clamping, and immediate removal of the placenta by cord traction.

☐ Physiological management entails allowing time for the cord to stop pulsating before clamping only the baby's end of the cord, letting blood drain into a bowl from the placental section, keeping the mother upright, and allowing her to deliver the placenta and membranes herself by pushing.

These two methods should never be mixed. To do so may provide a recipe for a retained placenta and postpartum haemorrhage.

Until the placenta separates from the uterine wall there is no bleeding and, even though the placenta may remain in the uterus for a long time, this is not dangerous. Your midwife or doctor may press in above your pubic bone and push upwards towards your navel to see if the cord moves up as the uterus is tipped upwards. If it does, the placenta is still attached *and no one should pull on the cord*, or it may cause bleeding. In hospitals sometimes an energetic attempt to complete the third stage results in the cord breaking. I have also known of women who have had the uterus pulled right down in this way.

The husband of a woman who gave birth without any assistance once phoned me to announce a happy birth three hours before and asked, "When should we expect the placenta?" I advised him to call a midwife, which he declined to do because the local health authority had refused to allow them a home birth. So I suggested that he help his wife into an upright position and, if the placenta did not fall out, that she should remain kneeling and put her lips around the stem of a bottle and give a long blow into it. She did this and the placenta dropped out. Among native women in South America this is a well-established practice to free a retained placenta. As air is exhaled, the abdominal press comes into play so that the mother's abdominal muscles press on her fundus and propel the placenta down. This is far safer than heaving the uterus around manually or tugging on the cord.

Postpartum haemorrhage

Occasionally a placenta does not peel away completely, and blood seeps from gaping sinuses in the muscle wall of the uterus. This is postpartum haemorrhage. It is more likely to occur after the uterus has been stretched with a twin pregnancy or with excess amniotic fluid, when a woman has haemorrhaged with a previous birth, following a difficult labour, or where there has been "fundus fiddling" by an anxious attendant. Elizabeth Davis says: "Left to itself the uterus will clamp down uniformly and will sheer off the placenta in one smooth sweep. But if poked and prodded may only release in certain sections."*

With postpartum haemorrhage the mother's blood pressure drops. Especially in poor countries many women are anaemic and cannot afford a heavy blood loss. Elizabeth Davis recommends that a woman in poor health in late pregnancy should have supplementary B vitamins (100 mg daily), plenty of protein- and iron-rich foods, and alfalfa tablets. Alfalfa is rich in vitamin K which facilitates clotting of blood.*

The first thing for the midwife or doctor to do if there are signs of haemorrhage is to give an intravenous injection of syntometrine and, if necessary, press the uterus firmly between two hands. A woman bleeds only if her uterus is soft and spongy and does not contract. It should be firm to the touch. If it is not, someone should massage it to stimulate it to contract. You can do this yourself, pressing in as if you are squeezing meringue mixture through an icing nozzle. Nipple stimulation, either from the baby breastfeeding, or done manually, also keeps the uterus firm. Once the uterus is firm and contracting, adopt a squatting or all-fours position, and the placenta should be delivered by steady, controlled cord traction with you in this position.

When the placenta is delivered, your doctor or midwife will check your pulse and blood pressure and may ask you to continue massaging the uterus to keep it well-contracted. They will stay with you for the next two hours or so.

Nowadays a healthy woman with high haemoglobin in pregnancy can cope with blood loss without having reduced haemoglobin afterwards. All the same, after a bleed it is sensible to take supplementary iron, and to eat iron-rich foods such as chocolate, eggs, molasses, dried fruits, watercress, and other green leafy vegetables. A blood test will be done a few days later to check your haemoglobin level.

"This delivery was so much exactly what a birth should be like, and it made such a strong impression and has given me such an 'easy', confident person of a baby, that I shall always be grateful . . . . It wasn't an earth-shattering experience but almost the opposite – a simple, straightforward event that happened naturally as part of the rhythm of the day."

The sudden, dramatic dash to hospital, sirens screaming; the grey and floppy baby who is barely breathing; the woman haemorrhaging massively – these fears are in the back of all our minds. But, because labour at home and in small GP units or alternative birth centres does not suffer the aggressive intervention to which many hospital labours are subjected, these are extremely rare events.

A carefully planned and lovingly conducted home birth, in which the rhythms of nature are respected and the woman is nurtured by attendants who have the knowledge and understanding to support the spontaneous unfolding of life, is the safest kind of birth there is, and the most deeply satisfying for everyone involved.

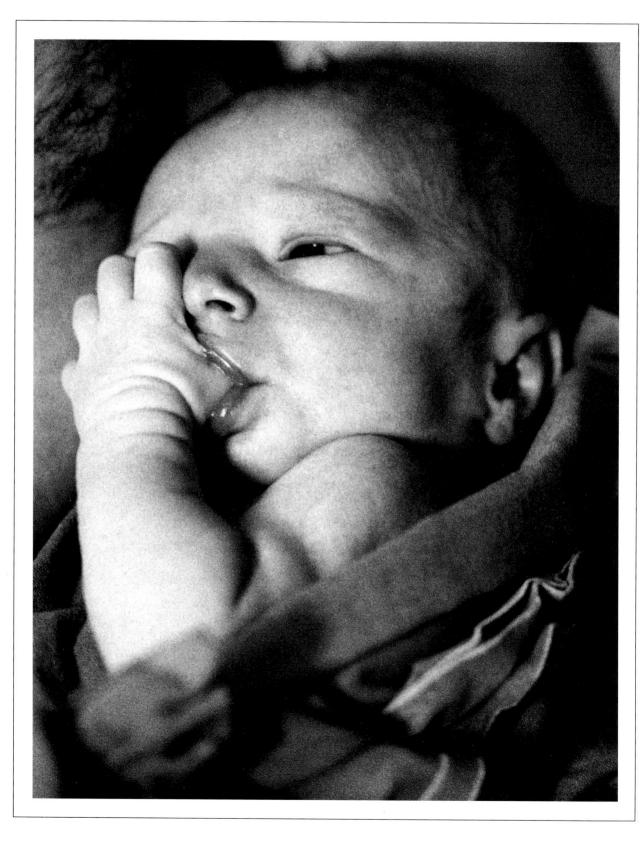

10

Birthways

There is no single ideal birth. There is instead the birth you have, the experience that is uniquely yours. With the support of friends who are sensitive to your needs, quick to respond to your wishes, who are emotionally nurturing, and who above all believe in you and your ability to give birth, childbirth can be an adventure in physical sensation and intense emotion, a journey of discovery of your own inner power that is exhilarating, sensuous and satisfying. This is how three very different women experienced birth in their own homes.

MANDY'S HOME BIRTH

This was Mandy's second baby. She had two birth companions: Nick, her partner, and Carly, a woman friend, who had special responsibility for Phoebe, her five-year-old. Labour started with a show at midday. Mandy went to collect Phoebe after school and took her swimming. Around 5 p.m. she felt certain that she was in labour, but contractions were mild and she couldn't tell when each one began or ended.

"Nick changed into cotton shorts and T-shirt because it was hot. By 5.50 p.m. I had started slow, deep, relaxing breathing during contractions, and he rubbed my back with massage oil."

"Phoebe came in from time to time. That was lovely. She gave me a kiss and a cuddle to reassure herself that we were still there and that we were all right. Nick's presence was very important to me. The midwives were lovely, but very much background figures."

Mandy made singing, moaning sounds with each long breath out. She stood up, leaning on Nick.

A midwife listened to the baby's heart regularly. A gas and oxygen mask was in the room, but Mandy didn't need it.

When Mandy stood, she felt dizzy because she had forgotten to eat lunch that day. The midwives suggested that she drink apple juice and suck glucose tablets because there were ketones in her urine. She did this and soon felt better. Mandy had explained that she wanted to cope with pain by using breathing and relaxation, and by bathing and keeping mobile, and that she would like an unhurried second stage. Her midwives were happy with this. For much of the time she was on all fours, or kneeling upright on the bed with her arms round Nick's neck. Later she knelt on the floor in front of a sofa, resting her head on the cushion, while he rubbed her back.

*"Then there was a catch in my breathing through each of
three contractions. Nick suggested that I squat up on the
sofa so that the midwife could examine me easily. I was
fully dilated – and could push. I kept my mouth wide open
during contractions and held on to Nick beside me."*

"The second stage was very intense, with virtually no gaps between contractions. I made a noise. I don't know how I could have given birth without using sound. They said, 'The head is coming. It's crowned.' We had a mirror. It was tremendously exhilarating!"

Mandy squatted on the sofa, her elbows on the back of it.

She reached down and gently touched the baby's head.

"I said, 'I want to touch it.' They said, 'That's fine.' I felt a little head, soft, warm, and wet, and there was a rush of falling in love with the baby. Then he was born. Nick helped me pull up my T-shirt so that the baby could snuggle against my body."

She breathed her baby out, without an episiotomy or a tear, and the cord was clamped only after it had stopped pulsating. It was 8.40 p.m., and evening sun was flooding in through the window.

The baby was covered in vernix. Mandy didn't notice what sex he was at first. It didn't seem important. A midwife handed the cord to Nick and said, "Tell us when you'd like to cut it," and he cut the cord.

"They helped me wrap him up in soft winceyette. He cried a bit. He wasn't particularly interested in the breast, but gave it the occasional lick. Then Nick held him while they delivered the placenta, without need of syntometrine. It slithered out five minutes after the birth."

The GP arrived and checked the baby.

"I felt so fortunate! This was an experience that I can always take out of my head and contemplate with pleasure and then put back in again. It made me feel enormously confident about myself and more confident in my mothering abilities. It was the best thing ever!"

Two minutes after the baby was born Mandy's friend brought Phoebe to meet him. She was quiet, in awe at the mystery of birth. The setting sun shone into the bedroom, lighting up Mandy's red-gold hair. The atmosphere was very calm and peaceful. Afterwards they all agreed that they felt tired, not only because of the hard physical work of birthing, but because of the high degree of emotion experienced in such a short space of time. The midwives thanked Mandy for allowing them to share her birth experience. They told her that they loved home births, which were a challenge to their training and enabled them really to practise as midwives.

Mandy felt fulfilled and elated. Phoebe gazed in wonder at the baby in her arms.

"The best thing about it was being at home and with my family. I was aware of a surge of endorphins about three hours before I gave birth. That was great! It was like dreaming. I could let go."

SIEGRUN'S HOME BIRTH

It was Siegrun and Vincent's first baby. Stephen, Vincent's brother, and Sarah, his partner, were the birth companions. They had come to stay some days earlier, and it seemed a long wait before labour started. The couple prepared together for the birth with meditation and massage, and by practising squatting positions. Siegrun was on all fours for most of her labour. Sarah knelt in front of her so that Siegrun could bury her head in her lap while Vincent held her back. The labour started at 11.30 a.m., and the baby was born at 4.10 p.m. after Siegrun had been pushing for only ten minutes.

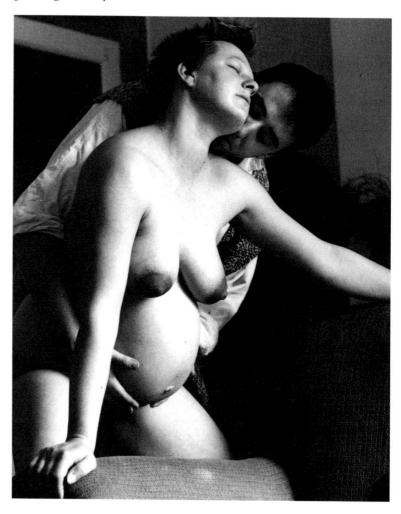

Siegrun felt strong and in touch with her feelings.

Everything seemed timeless, and pain was "in another dimension".

The pain she felt was low down by her cervix.

"The pushing was good. I couldn't push lying on my back, so I rolled over on to my side and said to Vincent, 'Hold my foot.' As I took in a breath, I took in life. I had two very strong pushes. I felt her head with my hands. There were two or three more pushes and the burning started. I said, 'I can't get it out.' Vincent said, 'We must have gravity on our side.' He lifted me and, as I got up, the baby shot out and the midwife caught her."

Her partner gave her strong, loving support.

As Vincent raised Siegrun into an upright position, the baby tumbled out very quickly, before anyone was quite ready for her. She was vigorous and healthy. The midwife clamped and cut the cord immediately, although Siegrun wanted to wait until it stopped pulsating.

"I heard a little scream, a noise like a cat, and realized that she was actually there. I'd forgotten that there would be a baby – Sarah said, 'It's a girl!' and I thought, 'Oh, God! I haven't got a girl's name!'"

"I started shivering. I put her straight to my breast, but it felt strange. I needed a little breathing space to lie back, close my eyes, and get back into myself before being able to give her everything she needed. Then the whole world was suddenly newborn. Something changed in me and in the world."

Overwhelmed with joy and wonder, Vincent took Siegrun in his arms and kissed her, their newborn baby clasped between them.

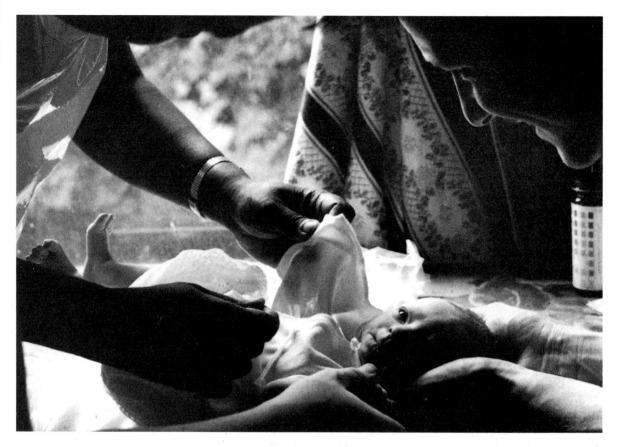

"Beforehand I was worried about the birth as a test of me and our relationship. When it came to it, it was so easy, so natural! I knew what to do."

Opposite "Siegrun was too freaked-out to hold the baby straight away, so I held her – tentatively at first, but I soon became confident. The experience has made me really close to our baby."

The midwife weighed the baby, cradled in a spring scale.

TESS'S WATER BIRTH

The relationship between Tess and her midwife was warm and close. Lesley did not interfere in any way, or offer advice, but simply waited quietly and gave her undivided attention.

Below Sometimes she squatted, holding the edge of the pool, and often she dipped and flipped over like a dolphin.

Below right Afternoon light streamed through the parted curtains, shining into the water, so that it was easy to catch the first glimpse of the baby's head as it pressed down.

My daughter Tess gave birth to her first child in a pool in our home. Our family GP did not wish to be involved, and told Tess that she was "high risk' because of her age (29) and because it would take half an hour to drive to the hospital, should the need arise. So two midwife friends, Lesley and Chloe, looked after Tess. One night Tess had backache and she decided to relax in the pool. She realized she was in labour the moment she stepped out of it at 1 a.m. and woke us at 4 a.m. when she wanted some support.

From 7.30 a.m. till midday she was partly walking in the garden, squatting and holding on to a tree when a contraction came, partly in my study. She leaned over a low birth stool, rested on all fours over cushions, or knelt or squatted, held by her helpers, the two midwives, Jon her husband, and myself. But she was so much more comfortable in the water that she jumped back into the pool, and remained in it for five hours. She sometimes lay back and floated. At other times she squatted. Her breathing was unforced and gentle, and she said that she forgot everything she learned in antenatal classes because it just came naturally.

She felt in a heightened state of self-awareness and inner confidence, and did not want to be fussed with either instructions or encouragement. She asked us all to keep quiet so that she could concentrate. The atmosphere was peaceful.

Once the head was born, Tess suddenly flipped over and knelt. Lesley delivered the baby's posterior shoulder first and he slid out. Tess needed no episiotomy and did not have a tear. Sam weighed 4.75 kg (10½ lb).

"I didn't like pushing the head round past my anus, but once it was on my perineum it felt much more purposeful. It was a happy sort of pain and I reached down and felt my baby's head. After the head was born the next contraction wasn't very strong and I lay back and relaxed for several minutes. Then a strong contraction came and I felt I needed to kneel forward, holding on to the side of the pool, so without thinking about it I just flipped over. Apparently this was the right thing to do, as he had broad shoulders."

"Lesley told me to give several big pushes. This was the hardest part of the birth in terms of sheer effort, but I wasn't aware of any pain. Then just one more push and he was born. I knelt up, turned towards Lesley, stepped over the cord, and reached out for my baby. He didn't cry, but I knew he was fine because you could see his strong muscles as he hugged himself and kicked. He didn't look anything like a newborn alien being. He was Sam."

*"I said 'Hello Sam' and he looked straight at me. He was so alert
and had such bright eyes! I could feel him breathing gently and
evenly. I just kept saying 'You're lovely! You've got chubby
cheeks.' He glanced around at the other people. Then, as I spoke
to him, he looked up at me and smiled. I held him close to my
breast, but he was not interested in sucking yet."*

"I had already decided that I didn't want to share the pool with a placenta. We cuddled in the water until Lesley said the cord had stopped pulsating. She wondered how I was going to get out, but I just stepped out. It was simple. I'd never felt better."

"I sat on a low stool and they wrapped us in soft, warm towels. Then the cord was cut and I held him close, and we marvelled at him and the whole miracle of birth. We were all so high the champagne was nice, but I don't think it added much to the occasion."

Tess never had any goal in her mind about having a water birth. She used water for pain relief and to help her centre down and let her body do the birth work. She waited to see how she felt at the time about actually giving birth in water. In the event, it seemed the most natural thing for her to stay in the water for the birth, as it also was natural to lift the baby out of the water and into her welcoming arms immediately he was born. She is quite sure that if she has another baby she will want to give birth in water again.

11

Babymoon

The time immediately following birth is precious. It should never deteriorate to being merely a sequel to delivery, an interval for postpartum recovery, or the kind of "bonding" time in which you feel you must fall in love with the baby fast or you are being an inadequate mother. In birth we have the opportunity ourselves to be reborn, to see the world with new clarity, and to experience life with an intensity that may otherwise be forgotten. A child is born, and for a moment the wheeling planets seem to stop in their tracks, as past, present and future meet. This sense of the miraculous, of incarnation and transcendence, often floods in wherever a baby is born. But when a woman is in her own space, when a couple feel at home in the environment in which they meet this new life, there is a special radiance. Being in a place that you control yourselves means that you need not conform to any standards, be self-consciously on your best behaviour, or worry about what other people are thinking of you. Instead, you are free to focus entirely on the baby.

PLANNING YOUR BABYMOON

The babymoon is the old "confinement" in contemporary idiom, adapted to the needs of a woman who, instead of having an extended family, experiences the deepest closeness with her sexual partner. It is a special time in the growth of love, and for many couples has a significance greater than that of the honeymoon, with consequences that may be long-lasting. The idea is simply that the couple create a setting in which they are intimately alone with their baby, and can get to know her without the intrusion of the usual responsibilities and social contacts. Your midwife calls in each day at first, to check on you and the baby, but otherwise you limit other people to a set visiting time, so that your intimacy is not invaded. All the baby-admiring and cuddling and cups of tea and sips of champagne can take place with friends and relatives sitting on and around the bed. At other times you have a note on the door that reads: "Please do not disturb. Mother and baby resting."

Unless you already have a child, and would welcome someone close to you who can give extra attention to the other child while you get to know your baby, this means putting off having your mother to stay, for example, till the end of this week or ten days, or however long you want the babymoon to last. It also entails careful planning ahead so that your partner can take time off work and you have food in store. If you have a freezer, you can shop and cook well ahead of time. Even if you don't, ensure that the cupboards are full. Before you start labour, buy plenty of fruit juices and other drinks, since breastfeeding makes you thirsty.

"It was well after two o'clock on Christmas morning. It was slightly snowing outside and Naomi was peacefully nursing at my breast. We celebrated for another couple of hours before everybody left to get ready for their Christmas celebrations at home."

Your partner will have to be chef, housekeeper, and butler, unless you are going to rely entirely on take-away meals and let the dirty dishes pile up. The phone is bound to ring a lot. Work out together how you want to deal with that. As well as time to cuddle, you will want time to sleep.

LYING IN

Traditionally women have always had a "lying in" time, a period of seclusion in which they could concentrate on the new baby and be cared for by other women. Although in situations of extreme poverty, war or famine, it is impossible to ensure this, it remains the ritual ideal in many cultures, and is a powerful functional bond in women's domestic culture.* The 40 days after birth are a time when the new mother is exempt from at least some of her usual tasks, and she receives special consideration, nourishing foods, and loving support from other women of the household, as she passes over the bridge into motherhood. Many of these women stay in the new mother's home for days or weeks afterwards.

During the earliest part of this period she is in an enclosed space, sometimes a darkened room, and access to outsiders is severely restricted. For she is in a marginal social and spiritual state, and she and the baby are considered to be especially vulnerable and tender.

Within traditional Judaic culture the new mother was cared for entirely by other women for the first 30 days after birth. They built a fire by her and this was fed even on the Sabbath, when such work was normally forbidden, and she was plied with sugary teas and nourishing food.

Usually the time of intensive loving care is shorter than this. In Fiji, for example, the new mother is tended by both of the grandmothers with two young women from her own kin group and two from the father's until the tenth day. In all traditional cultures there are nurturing women to help care for the new baby, take over household tasks such as cleaning and washing, and perhaps massage both mother and baby. They pride themselves on producing especially sustaining foods. In parts of India, for example, they prepare a drink of sweet coconut milk mixed with dill seed, which is thought to give the mother strength.

In today's industrial society, women are often expected to take over cooking and cleaning and caring for their husbands and other children, and to demonstrate that they have "got their figures back", within a few weeks, and sometimes mere days, after birth. They want to "return to normal", as if nothing has happened. It is all supposed to take place without a second thought, and with tremendous *joie de vivre*. Yet if a new mother is to be able to nurture her child, she herself needs to be nurtured. Most women need space and time, and cherishing from those closest to them, to make the major adjustment to motherhood, and the focus should be on neither recovery nor return, but rather on transformation.

If you are having your baby at home, or if you are returning home soon after the birth – the usual arrangement if you have your baby in a birth centre – my suggestion is that you may enjoy postpartum "nesting" in a king-sized bed. The whole focus of the home switches to the bed with its new life. It is as if, for a short space, your bed becomes the household shrine.

"This is when birth at home is so wonderful. You can sleep if and when you want, have the light on to look at your baby when you want, eat and drink when you want. Your husband and children are with you, and everybody can feel uninhibited in greeting and responding to the new baby at their own pace."

"I couldn't help grieving a little. It felt so magical to have her inside me. I had a feeling of emptiness when she was born. She was beautiful, but different from how I had imagined."

WELCOMING YOUR BABY

When a woman first meets her baby, she says goodbye to the fantasy baby inside her and greets the real one in her arms. This can be a difficult transition for a woman who had a clear idea that the baby was of one sex

"I knew instantly that she was mine. But there was an odd detachment too. It was as if there were two babies, and the baby inside me was retreating from me while Imogen was coming towards me. Part of me mourned that dark, mysterious baby inside me. At the same time I looked at Imogen and thought, 'We've arrived! Here is my family. Now this house is full of children, and that's how I want it to be.'"

and it turns out to be of the other, or who was sure that the baby would be perfectly formed and a handicap is revealed, or who expected that the baby would look like her or her partner, or be smaller or larger, or more attractive, than it actually is. A woman strives to find continuity of experience between the baby inside and the baby outside her body. It is not just that she needs time to come to terms with this reality. She may also need a sanctuary in which she can experience safely a range of conflicting emotions. A hospital is a difficult place in which to do this, with all its comings and goings, the routines of a large institution, and the social isolation from those closest to her that is often imposed on the new mother while she remains a "patient".

For many women who have their babies in hospital bonding is delayed and hindered, or sometimes never gets going, until after they are home, and occasionally not even then. New mothers tell of the frustration, demoralization, and depression at feeling caught up in an alien and threatening system that they are powerless to influence in any way, either for themselves or for their babies. They say such things as: "The nurses were liable to take the babies away with no explanation, and were surprised when asked what they were about to do"; "I felt like one of the cogs in a machine, not a person at all"; and "The mothers seemed to be there for them, and not the other way round."

Hospital staff may consider that the new mother's prime need is for rest, and want to ensure that each woman has uninterrupted sleep at night and rest-times during the day apart from her baby. In some hospitals, for example, babies born at night tend to be sent to the special care nursery even though they are perfectly all right, because it is the easiest thing to do, and it avoids disturbing other mothers.

One result of awareness of the importance of bonding, and of failure to bond being viewed as a cause of child abuse, is that in some hospitals nurses are on the look-out for potential child abusers. Sometimes mothers are acutely aware that they are under critical observation to reveal if they are responding appropriately to their babies. One woman, whose baby suffered from facial palsy, said, "They thought I was in danger of rejecting the baby," and she felt that they thrust him at her. Every time she went to the special care baby unit she felt that she had to put on a performance, and so began to avoid visiting it. The staff's enthusiasm to promote bonding actually made it more difficult for this woman to accept her baby.

Only in a warm, loving, and intimate environment can a woman feel secure in expressing her real emotions. Mothering grows from genuine feelings and bears no resemblance to the magazine image of a glamorous

"I felt my whole body and consciousness expand and fill with pleasure. At that moment I felt that I had been the agent of a miracle, had brought about a revelation not of a truth, but of a life, and with it immense humility and gratitude."

mother in a frilly negligée proudly cradling her new baby. When a woman becomes a mother, she may be swept along as if on a roller-coaster of fierce, passionate, and often conflicting emotions. Her identity as the mother of this particular child is forged not only through pleasure in her baby, but also through the anxiety, pain, and other negative feelings which stem naturally from the "primary maternal preoccupation" that is a normal accompaniment to falling in love with a baby.*

To carry a child in your body, to plan ahead, to make choices between alternatives, to give birth and hold your child in your arms is an experience that can bring with it profound emotional commitment, deep acceptance of responsibility, and a maturing of personality. It is not a medical event. It is a major life transition.

When you greet your baby on your own territory, those who help you come as guests, not guardians of medical space. The whole obstetric system is designed to control women, to render them passive, and to screen, treat, and regulate their reproductive functions for their own good. But in your space there are no rules to be obeyed, no standards to which you must conform. You are free to be yourself.

Lying together in bed with your baby, you and your partner both have extended time to explore the astonishing reality and the wonder of this new little being. You relive the experience of birth, learn how to respond to his signals, and can start breastfeeding at your own pace and in your own way. Your older children may enjoy cuddling in with you for some of the time, and at other times will need a loving person who can focus on their needs and enable you to have this special time with your baby.

You feel his plump firmness in your arms, stroke the down on the head, and see bright eyes gazing up at you. There is an excitement about breastfeeding that is going well. It is partly the *conviction* that you can meet your baby's needs, that your body is working well, that you can both give life and sustain it; partly the sensual *physical contact* and pleasurable holding and the surge of the milk flow, and partly the pre-verbal *conversation* with this small human being in your arms, as you get to know a wide-eyed creature for whom the whole world is new, who comes to you out of its raw, elemental being and turns to you in trust.

You will both become aware of your baby's rhythms, the cycles of sleep and waking, the times when he is alert, other times when he is fretful or drowsy, and the highpoints of his life, when he wakes hungry and discovers the firm sweetness of his mother's breasts and sucks avidly until he falls asleep, replete and utterly satisfied. You will enjoy "conversations" with your baby when he is in an awake and alert state. A baby is not merely at the receiving end of stimuli. He can communicate with you by his attention, the steady gaze of his eyes, his restlessness, or the glazed expression that comes on his face before he falls asleep at last. Parents don't need code books to understand this. All they require is unhurried time with their baby in an environment where they can act with spontaneity and are not inhibited by anybody else's expectations or theories. It is an environment that hospitals find very difficult to provide. But it exists already. It is home.

AN EMOTIONAL TRANSFORMATION

There is emotional work to be done too. The change from woman to mother occurs as if by grace, by enchantment, but it is also fraught with pain. When you have a baby, your view of the world changes. You see people, and other people's children, with new eyes. You become more vulnerable, more touched by suffering, more sensitively aware of need. You may weep more readily, be distressed by items on news programmes, feel bonded not only with your baby, but with all human beings, all living things, in a different way. Your whole relationship with time changes, and is moulded around your child's need of you. You often feel that time stretches out endlessly like a long ribbon with no end in sight. However it is, you cannot go on as before. Life has a new shape.

The transformation of woman to mother often has to occur in isolation from that of man to father, and as a result is qualitatively entirely different. After they have a child, many couples find that they each speak a different language and have widely divergent concerns. The mother is child-focused. The father is work-focused. This often happens even when the woman has a career, and up until now has had work at the centre of her life. A man may see a new baby as a possession, but for a woman the child is her flesh. Thus her identity is changed fundamentally, while his is not. You both need a space in your lives to pass through the transformation into being parents, to adjust together to the nakedness of feelings, the new fluidity of time, and the new centre to your lives.

YOUR OTHER CHILDREN

"My other two children saw her within minutes. For them birth is a normal process which can happen in the next bedroom, not a dark technological mystery."

If you already have a child, this oasis in time is one that nurtures your older child too. She also has to pass through a transformation, from special and only one to older sister, from baby to child. This process of growth cannot be rushed. She, too, needs time and a sanctuary. If your bed is big enough, she can cuddle up with you and the new baby, assured of your love for her, able to get to know the baby in her own way. Keep special playthings and story books close by, and have some favourite snacks handy. She won't want to stay with you long, but will bounce off to play, make things, have an adventure. Your partner will be kept busy coping with your older child's needs as well as yours. This kind of babymoon has a different flavour!

THE START OF BREASTFEEDING

Women can breastfeed against amazing odds. I have been in hospitals in the USSR where mothers are not handed their babies until four hours or longer after birth, by which time nurses have already swaddled them, and where women must have their fingers painted with iodine before they can touch their babies. Yet they breastfeed successfully – because they know they can, and the alternative of artificial feeding is not readily available.

Breastfeeding in hospital

The average hospital environment provides the worst possible start for breastfeeding. In spite of all the lip-service paid to breastfeeding in Britain, for example, in 30 per cent of big hospitals with consultant units women still cannot as a matter of course put their babies to the breast at birth. In 40 per cent of hospitals babies do not "room-in" with their mothers all the time, and 16 per cent of hospitals allow babies to be with their mothers only in the day-time.*

Babies are separated from their mothers "so that you can rest," "so that the baby isn't over-stimulated," "so as not to disturb the other mothers," "so that we can keep an eye on him," "because there is a rule that the baby must be in the nursery for the first two nights, and your milk hasn't come in, so there is no point in having him with you," or "because the baby is slightly jaundiced and needs phototherapy."

Hospitals are noisy places and in some sedatives are given routinely at night to all mothers, including those who are breastfeeding. One woman commented, "Going without a sleeping tablet seems to be regarded as a perversion." Crying babies are often whisked away to the nursery, and may be given formula by nurses who try to keep the ward peaceful, and who may also enjoy the chance to feed and look after the babies.

Only 30 per cent of hospitals give no additional fluids to breastfed babies: 25 per cent offer water if they think the baby needs it, 7 per cent offer it routinely, and 38 per cent give the babies glucose solution and/or artificial milk.*

"It was good that my mum had the baby in the holidays because I was so excited that I did not get to sleep until three o'clock in the morning. For a whole week we had dinner in my mum's room with champagne. Like a picnic to celebrate."
An older sister

Women are the target of a great deal of conflicting advice from different caregivers too. They often feel that they have to show that they are following the advice given by whoever is watching them at the time, and as a result become bewildered and disheartened. They sometimes comment that although usually capable and self-assured, they seemed especially vulnerable in hospital, and were surprised at how easily they felt put down or humiliated.

There is general approval of "demand feeding" in many hospitals. Yet even within the same hospital, there may be different interpretations of what this actually is. Many nurses see it as feeding whenever the baby cries, *but* not more often than every two hours or less often than every five hours. In some hospitals mothers are encouraged to follow their babies' lead but must fill in forms indicating when they have fed. They often find it difficult to do this in a relaxed and spontaneous way because, as one said, "I felt inhibited about owning up to each nibble of colostrum." As a result they "cheat" on the charts, and give the impression that the baby is suckling less often than is the case.*

Regulations to keep other staff members happy, including doctors, ward cleaners, and caterers, or to present the ward as an orderly, well-managed place to visitors, often restrict feeding-times to certain hours. So mothers may be told that they must not feed at meal-times, during ward cleaning, at rest-times, during the physiotherapy exercise session, during doctors' ward rounds, when they should be having a bath, and at visiting times. As one woman said, "The hospital seemed to treat babies' feeding-times as a necessary evil interrupting hospital routine." As a result babies cry a lot. An Asian mother in a London hospital, wondering at the strange way in which Europeans seem to treat their babies, asked, "Why do the English punish their babies?"

The most usual reasons that are cited for giving up breastfeeding are "insufficient milk", that the baby "rejected the breast or failed to latch on", and "sore nipples".*

Some nurses approve of breastfeeding if it comes easily, but expect mothers to switch to artificial feeding if there are problems, and to stay relaxed about it. They often give tireless devotion, sitting with women to help them establish breastfeeding, but some do not understand the skills of breastfeeding and the art of encouraging a baby to latch on. They are also concerned that emphasis on breastfeeding makes those mothers who are advised to feed artificially feel that they are failures, and seem to hope for a slightly detached attitude in the mother. One woman who resisted the suggestion that her baby should be artificially fed wrote, "Sister said she had

"Ally was very tired after the birth but, because she was at home, she could rest. If she had been forced to adapt to a hospital routine, I think she would have been utterly exhausted."
A father

expected trouble with me because I was 'one of those mothers who are determined to breastfeed, come what may'."

It is not surprising that in Britain 19 per cent of first-time mothers and 15 per cent of all mothers have stopped breastfeeding even before they leave hospital, and that by the end of the sixth week after birth only 38 per cent are still breastfeeding, and at four months only 26 per cent.* Nearly half of all breastfed babies have artificial milk supplements within their first week of life. By the end of the second week 28 per cent of those babies who had supplementary feeds are fed artificially, compared with only 8 per cent of those who had no supplementary feeds.

Your own space for breastfeeding

The joy of starting breastfeeding in your own environment is that you do not have to put on a demonstration to anyone or prove that you can do it successfully. Instead it is a secret and delightful conspiracy between you and the baby. Breastfeeding is a natural element in your developing relationship that is exciting and satisfying for you both, an adventure in sensation and touch, and in the gradual unfolding of personality of this new human being and this new mother. Breastfeeding is a way of communicating, a way of loving. Because this is so, it is never merely a matter of technique.

"I was given Hilary almost immediately while they dealt with the placenta. She suckled straight away. She was beautiful. When everyone had left and she had been put in her crib, she wouldn't settle, so I lifted her out and I lay nursing her for the rest of the night. Neither Duncan nor I had experienced such complete happiness ever before."

There may be pain mixed strangely with the tenderness and desire. As your baby's sucking stimulates contractions of the uterus, helping it to return almost to its pre-pregnant size and shape, your breasts become full, heavy, and swollen. When the baby latches on, you experience the urgency of the milk-ejection reflex, and your breasts become flushed and hot.

When you are in your own intimate place, a place that you have created, you realize that breastfeeding is not just a matter of what a woman does with her breasts, but rather of her sense of positive identity as a woman and a mother, and that when she breastfeeds an intense flow of energy surges through her whole body.

NIGHT NESTING

Even after your babymoon has finished, you can keep the same closeness if you have "night nesting". By this I mean that you have your baby sleeping in bed with you instead of in a cot. Traditionally mothers have always slept with their babies, and still do so in many cultures, even in the highly evolved industrial society of Japan. In contrast, Western emphasis on children's development of autonomy – being independent and achieving –

"Demand feeding was easy because I had the baby in bed with me."

dictates that a baby should be in his own cot, in his own room, and should not disrupt adult activities.

When you have your baby in bed with you, the physical closeness, the sounds of your breathing and beating heart, and the warmth of your body are comforting for your baby, and having the baby beside you to touch and to gaze at when you wish is reassuring for you. However busy and rushed you are during the day, night nesting ensures undisturbed time with your baby. You can breastfeed without really waking, and snuggle down with your baby falling asleep again still on your breast.

This is not dangerous. Healthy newborns move their heads away if their noses are obstructed, and are in no danger of being "overlaid", although it is wise not to have a baby in bed if either you or your partner has been drinking heavily or has taken drugs that reduce awareness. A really large bed with a firm mattress makes this arrangement more comfortable for all of you. However, there is also an advantage in accustoming the baby to sleeping separately sometimes too, so that later on you do not always have to go to bed every time you want your child to settle down.

If you are going back to work again soon after the birth, night nesting and breastfeeding whenever your baby wants to stimulates milk production, and means that you can continue breastfeeding even if your baby is being cared for by someone else for the major part of the day. You may have such a good milk supply that you need to express milk while you are at work lest you become engorged. You can do this simply with a small, portable electric pump, or even by hand if you are adept at it. Then you can store this milk in a refrigerator so that someone else can give it to the baby in a bottle.*

All over the world, in widely varying cultures, women breastfeed while at the same time working in and outside their homes, labouring in the fields, cracking stones to make roads, washing the family's clothing in the river, or gathering berries and other foods in the bush. They don't retire to bed or to a nursery to breastfeed. It is part of a busy life in which the baby's needs are met and the baby is breastfed wherever the mother happens to be. At night mother and baby cuddle in bed together, and the baby may suck on and off through the hours of darkness. This is a pattern of breastfeeding which has been highly successful, and it is one that women in industrial societies are now rediscovering for themselves.

EMOTIONS AFTER BIRTH

Nobody knows how many women suffer from depression after childbirth. In Western countries one in ten receives medical treatment for depression.*

Almost half of those treated are still depressed a year later. But this is just the tip of the iceberg. A great many women do not realize that they are depressed, and many of those who do have no help in dealing with their depression. New mothers often seek advice about breastfeeding difficulties, for example, yet are really asking for help with their own inturned anger and feelings of helplessness and worthlessness. Statistics of clinical depression do not include these distressed women.

Postnatal depression is often envisaged as a kind of mental fog that seeps out of a woman's bloodstream and reproductive organs. According to this view, nothing can be done to prevent it, and when it happens women are treated as if they are sick, may be prescribed mood-changing drugs, and be told that ultimately the cure lies within themselves. But, in fact, depression has specific *social* causes, and there may be many things in a woman's life that contribute to it.

Depression after the birth of a baby is less to do with the hormonal disturbance to which it is often attributed than to all the pressures on a woman to conform to the pattern of a happy new mother, to the socio-economic stresses on women who are living in poverty,* and, very often, to the experience of being disempowered by childbirth in hospital. My own research reveals that the institutional violence typical of care in many hospitals results in the depersonalization and disabling of women. As a result, some new mothers are left trying to cope with feelings that are very similar to those a woman experiences after being raped, and which often persist weeks, months, and even years later.

There is debate among psychologists and sociologists as to whether obstetric intervention in childbirth is associated with depression. Some research suggests that the more obstetric intervention takes place, the more women suffer from depression.* Certainly women are more likely to be depressed after Caesarean section.*

Women who feel that they were denied any control over what was done to them in childbirth are at greater risk of being unhappy in the week following birth than those who feel that they were in control.* It is not so much whether there is intervention, but a woman's sense of control or loss of control over what is being done to her, that is important.* This may be why women who have planned Caesarean sections are less likely to suffer postnatal depression than those who have unplanned Caesarean sections, when the decision is made once labour has started, often over their heads and over their supine bodies.*

Women who have suffered depression after a first baby sometimes decide to have the next birth at home because they are convinced that the hospital environment was in large measure responsible for their later emotional distress. There is mounting evidence that they are correct in their belief, and that a woman's feelings of wellbeing are enhanced when she is able to give birth in an environment that she herself controls. When you give birth in an environment of your own making – one that you yourself control – you are more likely to experience postnatal euphoria than postnatal depression.

I am not claiming that if you have your baby at home you will never feel unhappy, low, or unable to cope. This is part of the human condition. What I am suggesting is that pervading anxiety, panic attacks, loss of confidence, feelings of worthlessness, and an uneasy sense that the baby does not really belong to you and that you have no right to be a mother, are for many women a result of the way in which they are treated when they give birth in hospital. The disempowering of women during a major life transition is distressing not only at the time; it may have long-term emotional effects.

A woman who controls the space in which she gives birth, and who can therefore risk losing her self-control, and surrender to the feelings welling up inside her during birth, is more likely to look back on the birth as a positive experience, and is less vulnerable to depression than one whose autonomy has been destroyed, and who feels that she has been violated.

In an intimate, loving environment, the experience of birth can be empowering. Especially for any woman who is vulnerable to depression or violent mood swings, one with low self-esteem, or who has suffered sexual abuse, birth can be healing. Childbirth is then an adventure in which you discover your own inner strength, joy in your body, and your capacity to give life and to open yourself in love.

Postscript

Birth, like death, is a universal human experience that we share. It can be an interruption of life, a medical episode, a solitary trial of endurance, a surgical operation on a patient who relies entirely on the obstetric expertise of those caring for her, and a frightening process in which women are trapped by their biology. Or it can be lived through in beauty and dignity, as new life emerges cradled in love and caring. It can be a celebration of joy, which takes place in spite of pain. For the energy flooding through a woman's body in birth, although it brings pain as a side-effect, is life-enhancing and powerful.

Choosing their own birthplace – one in which they feel secure – creating a nest that meets the needs of the mother and her newborn, is something that all mammals do, unless, like animals in a zoo, they are in captivity.

Women in our post-industrial culture are effectively captive in childbirth. The zoo may be run on scientific principles, the keepers may be considerate and may pride themselves on the good condition of their animals and the low mortality rate. Visiting times may be frequent and the zoo may be a friendly, welcoming place. In the confines of the cage there may be space to move about, and those in charge may have tried to replicate the natural habitat. Yet captivity restrains and dictates the behaviour of the captives.

At present saying "no" to hospital, making an informed decision to give birth in a place of your own choosing, is for most of us the only way to reclaim the experience of childbirth for women.

There is a challenge facing the maternity services today over and above the basic requirement to make birth as safe as possible for mothers and babies. This challenge consists of two main issues. The first is to provide genuine choice. It must include the provision of a really good home birth service and, for those who prefer them, small GP units and alternative birth centres. The second important issue is to enable women giving birth in hospital to control the birthplace there, too, so that they are not merely at the receiving end of care, however kind and compassionate it may be.

When we affirm our freedom by making an informed choice between alternatives, and select a place where *we*, not the doctors, are in control, we have an opportunity to rediscover in ourselves the power to give birth without any intervention, with the same confidence and spontaneity with which we breathe and move, and with the same love and passion with which we may have conceived the child who now enters the world.

USEFUL CONTACT ADDRESSES

National Childbirth Trust (NCT)

England:
Alexandra House
Oldham Terrace
Acton
London W3 6NH
Tel: 081-992 8637

Scotland:
2 Circus Gardens
Edinburgh EH3 6TN
Tel: 031-225 6847

Northern Ireland:
See *England*, above

Irish Childbirth Trust

Dublin:
Sue Jameson
66 Terenure Road East
Rothgar
Dublin 6
Tel: Dublin 909 795

Cork:
Deirdre Martin
82 Earlwood Estate
Cork
Tel: Cork 968 202

The Home Birth Centre

c/o The Mews
4 Leinster Road
Rathmines
Dublin 6
Tel: Dublin 977 342

AIMS (Association for Improvements in the Maternity Services)

England:
Sandar [sic] Warshal
40 Kingswood Avenue
London NW6 6LS
Tel: 081-960 5585

Scotland:
Nadine Edwards
40 Leamington Terrace
Edinburgh EH10 4JL
Tel: 031-229 6259

Northern Ireland:
Vicki McGlade
32 South Parade
Ormeau Road
Belfast 7
Tel: Belfast 644 354

Southern Ireland:
Maire O'Regan
18 Firgrove Drive
Bishopstown
Cork
Tel: Cork 342 649

Independent Midwives Association

65 Mount Nod Road
London SW16 2LP

ARM (Association of Radical Midwives)

62 Greetby Hill
Ormskirk
Lancashire L32 2DT
Tel: 0695 72776

Special Delivery Midwifery Practice

34 Elm Quay Court
Nine Elm Lane
London SW8 5DE
Tel: 071-498 2322
Private home birth service, antenatal care, classes, postnatal care for 4 weeks and mother's help for 2 weeks after birth; or help with arranging NHS home birth

Women's Health and Reproductive Rights Information Centre

52-54 Featherstone Street
London EC1Y 8RT
Tel: 071-251 6332/6580

Society to Support Home Confinement

Lydgate
Lydgate Lane
Wolsingham
Bishop Aukland
Co. Durham DL13 3HA
Tel: 09565 528044

Homebirth Movement

22 Anson Road
London N7 0RD

Maternity Alliance

15 Britannia Street
London WC1X 9JP
071-837 1273

La Lèche League of Great Britain

Box BM3424
London WC1N 3XX
Tel: 071-242 1278/071-404 5011

International Centre for Active Birth

55 Dartmouth Park Road
London NW5 1SL
Tel: 071-267 3006

Meet-a-Mum Association

5 Westbury Gardens
Luton
Bedfordshire LU2 7DW
Tel: 0582 422253

Gingerbread

35 Wellington Street
London WC2 7BN
Tel: 071-240 0953/0954

Arabella Marshall

18 Cistern Street
Totnes
Devon TQ9 5SP
Tel: 0803 863215

BIRTH POOLS

International Centre for Active Birth

Address as listed above

Birthworks

Hill House Community
Folleigh Lane
Long Ashton
Bristol BS19 9JB
Tel: Bristol 394202

Splashdown Birth Pools

Jayn and Richard Ingrey
68 West Street
Harrow on the Hill
Middlesex HA1 3ER
Tel: 081-422 9308

REFERENCES

These research references relate to the asterisks in the main text. Where there is more than one asterisk on a page, the references appear in order, with each entry on a new line relating to a different asterisk.

p. 11 Doering S., Entwistle D. (1975) "Preparation during pregnancy and ability to cope with labor and delivery", *American Journal of Orthopsychiatry*, 45, 825-837; Norr K., Block C., Charles A., Meyering S., Meyers E. (1977) "Explaining pain and enjoyment in childbirth", *Journal of Health and Social Behaviour*, 10, 260-275; Doering S., Entwistle D., Quinlan D. (1980) "Modeling the quality of women's birth experience", *Journal of Health and Social Behavior*, 21, 12-21; Entwistle D., Doering S. (1981) *The First Birth*, Baltimore: John Hopkins University Press; Romito P. (1989) "Unhappiness after childbirth", *Effective Care in Pregnancy and Childbirth*, 2, 1433-1446, eds. Chalmers I., Enkin M., Keirse M. J. N. C.; Kitzinger J. in Garcia J., Kilpatrick R., Richards M. (1990) *The Politics of Maternity Care*, Oxford: Clarendon Press; Kitzinger S., "Childbirth and violence against women", (forthcoming) *Women's Health Matters*, ed. Roberts H., London: Routledge.
□ Kitzinger S. (1987) *Some Women's Experiences of Epidurals*, London: National Childbirth Trust.

p. 18 Simkin P. (1986) "Stress, pain and catecholamines in labor: part 1, a review", *Birth*, 13, 4, 227-233.

p. 19 Association of Anaesthetists (1988) *Report on Obstetric Services*, London.

p. 20 Chalmers I., Richards M. P. M. (1977) "Intervention and causal inference in obstetric practice", *Benefits and Hazards of the New Obstetrics*, London: Heinemann, 34-61, eds. Chard T., Richards M. P. M.
□ Newcombe R. G., Chalmers I. (1977) "Changes in distribution of gestational age and birthweight among first-born infants of Cardiff residents", *British Medical Journal*, 2, 925-926; Chalmers I. et al (1978) "Respiratory distress syndrome in infants of Cardiff residents during 1965-1975", *British Medical Journal*, 2, 1119-1121; Newcombe R. G. (1983) "Reversal of changes in distribution of gestational age and birthweight among first-born infants of Cardiff residents", *British Medical Journal*, 287, 1095-1097.
□ MacFarlane A. J., Mugford M. (1984) *Birth Counts*, London: HMSO.
□ Cartwright A. (1979) *The Dignity of Labour?*, London: Tavistock.

p. 21 Kitzinger S. (1975) *Some Women's Experiences of Induced Labour*, London: National Childbirth Trust.

p. 22 O'Driscoll K., Meagher D. (1980) "Active management of labour", *Clinical and Obstetric Gynaecology* (supplement 1), ed. W. B. Saunders.
□ ibid.
□ ibid.

p. 23 ibid.
□ Taylor R. W., Taylor M. (1988) Letter to the *Lancet* 1, 8581, 352.
□ Placek P.J., Keppel K. G., Taffel S. M., Liss T. L. (1984) "Electronic fetal monitoring in relation to caesarean section delivery for live births and still births in the US 1980", *Public Health Reports*, 99, 173-183.
□ Nielson P. V., Stigsby B., Nickelson C., Nim J. (1987) "Intra- and inter-observer variability in the assessment of intrapartum cardiotocograms", *Acta Obstetricia et Gynecologia Scandinavica*, 66, 421-424.
□ Grant A. (1989) "Monitoring the fetus during labour", *Effective Care in Pregnancy and Childbirth*, 2, 846-882, Oxford: Oxford University Press, eds. Chalmers I., Enkin M., Keirse M. J. N. C.

p. 24 Macdonald D., Grant A., Sheridan-Pereira M., Boylan P., Chalmers I. (1985) "The Dublin randomized trial of intrapartum fetal heart rate monitoring", *American Journal of Obstetrics and Gynecology*, 152, 524-539.
□ ibid.; Grant A., (1987b) "The relationship between obstetrically preventable intra-partum asphyxia, abnormal neonatal neurological signs and subsequent motor impairment in babies born at or after term", *Perinatal Events and Brain Damage in Surviving Children*, Berlin: Springer Verlag, eds. Kubli F., Patel N., Schmidt W., Linderkamp O.
□ Amato J. G. (1983) "Fetal heart-rate monitoring", *American Journal of Obstetrics and Gynecology*, 147, 967-969.

□ Visser G. H. A., Goodman J. D. S., Dawes G. S. (1980) "Problems with ultrasonic fetal heart-rate monitor", *Lancet*, 1, 707-708.

p. 25 Sharp D. G., Couriel J. M. (1985) "Penetration of the subarachnoid space by fetal scalp electrode", *British Medical Journal*, 291, 1169.
□ d'Souza S. W. (1982) "Fetal scalp damage and neonatal jaundice: A risk of fetal scalp electrode monitoring", *International Journal of Obstetrics and Gynecology*, 2, 161-164.
□ Enkin M. (1989) "Labour and delivery following previous caesarean section", *Effective Care in Pregnancy and Childbirth*, 2, 1196-1217, eds. Chalmers I., Enkin M., Keirse M. J. N. C.

p. 27 Kitzinger S. (1989) "Perceptions of pain in home and hospital birth", Paper given at the International Congress of Psychosomatic Obstetrics and Gynaecology, Amsterdam.
□ Garcia J., Garforth S., Ayers S. (1986) "Midwives confined? Labour ward policies and routines", *Research and the Midwife Conference Proceedings*, University of Manchester, 74-78.

p. 28 Cohen W. R. (1977) "Influence of the duration of second stage labor on perinatal outcome and puerperal morbidity", *Obstetrics and Gynecology*, 49, 266-269.
□ Caldeyro-Barcia R. (1979) "The influence of maternal bearing-down efforts during second stage on fetal wellbeing", *Birth and the Family Journal*, 6, 17-21.

☐ Thacker S. E., Banta H. D. (1983) "Benefits and risks of episiotomy: An interpretive review of the English language literature, 1860-1980", *Obstetrical and Gynecological Survey*, 38, 322-338.

p. 29 ibid.; Sleep J. M., Grant A., Garcia J., Elbourne D., Spencer J., Chalmers I. (1984) "West Berkshire perineal management trial", *British Medical Journal*, 289, 587-590; Harrison R. F., Brennan M., North P. M., Reed J. V., Wickham E. A. (1984) "Is routine episiotomy necessary?", *British Medical Journal*, 288, 1971-1975; Sleep J. M., Grant A. (1987) "West Berkshire perineal management trail: Three year follow-up", *British Medical Journal*, 295, 749-751.
☐ Sleep J. M., Grant A., Garcia J., Elbourne D., Spencer J., Chalmers I., op. cit.; Harrison R. F., Brennan M., North P. M., Reed J. V., Wickham E. A., op. cit.
☐ Kitzinger S., Simkin P. (1990) *Episiotomy and the Second Stage of Labor*, Pennypress Inc.
☐ Kitzinger S., Walters R. (1981) *Some Women's Experiences of Episiotomy*, London: National Childbirth Trust.

p. 30 ibid.
☐ ibid.
☐ ibid.
☐ ibid.
☐ ibid.

p. 31 Davis E. (1981) *Heart and Hands*, California: Celestial Arts; Flint C. (1988) *Sensitive Midwifery*, London: Heinemann, 101-102.
☐ Cordero L., Hon E. (1971) "Neonatal bradychardia following nasopharyngeal stimulation", *Journal of Pediatrics*, 78, 441-447.

☐ Tyson J., Silverman W., Reisch J. (1989) "Immediate care of the newborn infant", *Effective Care in Pregnancy and Childbirth*, 2, 1293-1312, eds. Chalmers I., Enkin M., Keirse M. J. N. C.
☐ ibid.

p. 32 Cordero L., Hon E., op. cit.; Widstrom A.-M., Ransjo-Arvidson A. B., Christensson K., Matthieson A.-S., Winberg J., Uvnas-Moberg K. (1987) "Gastric suction in healthy newborn infants: Effect on circulation and developing feeding behaviour", *Acta Paediatrica Scandinavica*, 76, 566-572.
☐ Wahlberg V., Lundh W., Winberg J. (1982b) "Reconsideration of Crede prophylaxis III: Effects of silver nitrate prophylaxis on visual alertness in neonates", *Acta Paediatrica Scandinavica*, 295 (Supplement), 43-48; Wahlberg V., Lundh W., Winberg J. (1982c) Reconsideration of Crede prophylaxis IV: Effects of silver nitrate prophylaxis on mother infant relationship", *Acta Paediatrica Scandinavica*, 295 (Supplement), 49-57; Wahlberg V., Lundh W., Winberg J. (1982d) "Reconsideration of Crede prophylaxis V: Long-term influences on conjunctival secretion, infant behaviour, breastfeeding and maternal feelings. A descriptive study", *Acta Paediatrica Scandinavica* (Supplement) 59-67.
☐ Rothenberg (1979) "Ophthalmia neonatorum due to Neisseria gonorrhoeae: Prevention and treatment", *Sexually Transmitted Diseases*, 6 (Supplement), 187-190.
☐ Hammerschlag M. R., Chandler J. W., Alexander R., English M., Chiang W. T., Koutsky L., Eschenbach D. A., Smith J. R. (1980)

"Erythromycin ointment for ocular prophylaxis of neonatal chlamydial infection", *Journal of the American Medical Association*, 244, 2291-2293.
☐ Klaus M. H., Kennell J. H. (1982) *Parent Infant Bonding*, St Louis: C. V. Mosby, 56.
☐ World Health Organization (1985).

p. 35 Anderson S., Stangard F. (1986) *Traditional Midwives*, Goteborg: Ipelgang, 17-18.

p. 38 Chalmers I. (1990) "The risks and benefits of 'risk assessment' in childbirth", Speech at a forum on maternity and the newborn, London: Royal Society of Medicine.

p. 39 Mahmood T. A., Campbell D. M., Wilson A. W. (1988) "Maternal height, shoe size, and outcome of labour in white primigravidas: A prospective anthropometric study", *British Medical Journal*, 297, 515-517.

p. 40 Dickson Luce J. (1981) "Thoughts on 'risk'", *Maternal Health News*, 6, 4.

p. 41 Bastion H., Lancaster P. A. L. (1990) *Home Births in Australia 1985-1987*, Sydney: National Perinatal Statistics Unit.
☐ Tew M. (1985) "Place of birth and perinatal mortality", *Journal of the Royal College of General Practitioners*, 35, 390-394.

p. 42 Campbell R., Macfarlane A. (1990) "Recent debate on the place of birth", *The Politics of Maternity Care*, Oxford University Press, 217-237, eds. Garcia J., Kilpatrick R., Richards M.
☐ Social Security Committee (1980) *Perinatal and Neonatal Mortality* (second report), London: HMSO.

☐ Tew M. (1981) "Effects of scientific obstetrics on perinatal mortality", Health and Social Services Journal, 91, 444-446; Campbell R., Macdonald Davies I., Macfarlane A. (1982) "Perinatal mortality and place of delivery", *Population Trends*, 28, London: HMSO, 9-12; Campbell R., Macdonald Davies I., Macfarlane A., Beral V. (1984) "Home birth in England and Wales: Perinatal mortality according to intended place of delivery", *British Medical Journal*, 289, 721-724.
☐ Butler N., Bonham D., (1963) *Perinatal Mortality 1958*, London: Livingstone; Chamberlain R. *et al*, op. cit.; Tew M. (1990) *Safer Childbirth*, London: Chapman & Hall.
☐ Chamberlain R. *et al*, op. cit.

p. 43 Campbell R., Macfarlane A. (1987) *Where to be Born? The Debate and the Evidence*, Oxford: National Epidemiology Unit.
☐ Chamberlain R., Chamberlain G., Howlett B., Claireaux A. (1975) *British Births 1970*, London: Heinemann.
☐ Tew M. (1985) op. cit.
☐ Tew M. (1990) op. cit.
☐ ibid.

p. 44 ibid.
☐ ibid.
☐ Tew M. (1990) "Home birth: The issue of safety", Study day on home birth – exploring the issues, Birmingham Maternity Hospital: National Childbirth Trust.

p. 45 Wright J. T. (1983) "Alcohol and drug abuse in pregnancy", *Medicine International*, 35, 1630-1631.
☐ Calandra C., Abell D. A., Beischer N. A. (1981) "Maternal obesity in pregnancy," *Obstetrics and Gynecology*, 57, 8-12; Garbakiak J. A., Richter M., Miller S., Barton J. J. (1985) "Maternal weight and pregnancy

complications", *American Journal of Obstetrics and Gynecology*, 152, 238-245.
☐ Garbakiak J. A. *et al*, op. cit.
☐ Chamberlain R. *et al*, op. cit.; eds. James D. K., Stirrat G. M. (1988) *Pregnancy and Risk: The Basis for Rational Management*, Chichester: John Wiley & Sons.

p. 46 Bird C. (1971) "The premenopausal gravida", *Journal of Reproductive Medicine*, 6, 48-50.
☐ Kirz D. S., Dorchester W., Freeman R. K. (1985) "Advanced maternal age", *American Journal of Obstetrics and Gynecology*, 152, 1, 7-12.
☐ Cario G. M., Fray R. E., Morris N. F. (1985) "The obstetric performance of the elderly primigravida", *British Journal of Obstetrics and Gynecology*, 54, 237-240.

p. 47 Hofmeyr G. J. (1989) "Breech presentation and abnormal lie in late pregnancy", *Effective Care in Pregnancy and Childbirth*, 1, 635-666, Oxford: Oxford University Press, eds. Chalmers I., Enkin M., Keirse M. J. N. C.
☐ Hughey M. J. (1985) "Fetal position during pregnancy", *American Journal of Obstetrics and Gynecology*, 153, 885-886.
☐ Westgren M., Edvall H., Nordstrom E., Svalenius E. (1985) "Spontaneous cephalic version of breech presentation in the late trimester", *British Journal of Obstetrics and Gynecology*, 92, 19-22.

p. 48 Bakketeig L. S., Hoffman H. J. (1981) "Epidemiology of preterm birth: Results from a longitudinal study of births in Norway", *Preterm Labour*, London: Butterworth's International Medical Review, 17-40, eds. Elder M. G., Hendricks C. H.

☐ Salzmann B. (1964) "Rupture of low segment cesarean section", *American Journal of Obstetrics and Gynecology*, 23, 460-466.
☐ Beard R. W., Lowy C. (1986) "The British survey of diabetic pregnancies", *British Journal of Obstetrics and Gynaecology*, 89, 78326.

p. 49 James D. K., Stirrat G. M. eds., op. cit., 58.
☐ de Swiet M. (1986) "Pre-existing medical diseases", *Prepregnancy Care: A Manual for Practice*, Chichester: John Wiley & Sons, 69-111, eds. Chamberlain G., Lumley J.

p. 50 Taylor David J. *et al* (1985) "Do pregnancy complications contribute to neurodevelopmental disability?", *Lancet*, 1, 713-716.

p. 52 Steer P. (1988) "Risks in labour", *Pregnancy and Risk*, 6, 105-137, eds. James D. K., Stirrat G. M.

p. 62 Rooks P. J., Wetherby N. I., Ernst E. K. M., Stapleton S., Rosen D., Rosenfield A. (1989) "Outcome of care in birth centers", *New England Journal of Medicine*, 321, 26, 1804-1811.
☐ Eakins P. S. (1986) *Free-standing birth centers in California: Structure, Cost, Medical Outcome, and Issues*, Californian Department of Health Services.

p. 63 Feldman E., Hurst M. (1987) "A comparison of hospital and birth center settings", *Birth*, 18-24.
☐ Lumley J., Davey B. (1987) "Do hospitals with family-centered maternity care policies have lower intervention rates?", *Birth*, 132-134.
☐ Klein M. *et al* (1984) "Care in a birth room versus a conventional setting: A

controlled trial", *Canadian Medical Association Journal*, 131, 1461-1466.

p. 64 Chamberlain R. *et al*, op. cit.
☐ Rosenblatt R. A., Reinken J., Shoemack P. (1985) "Is obstetrics safe in small hospitals? Evidence from New Zealand's regionalized perinatal system", *Lancet*, 2, 429-432.

p. 65 Mugford M., Stilwell J. (1986) "Maternity services: how well have they done and could they do better?" *Health Care, Policy Journals*.

p. 67 Leicester Home Birth Support Group (February 1990) *Homebirth Newsletter*.

p. 74 Houd S. (1989) "Midwifery in some European countries", eds. van Hall E. V., Everaerd W., op cit.

p. 76 Barrington E. (1985) "Birth stories and midwives' musings", *Midwifery is Catching*, 101.
☐ Kirkham M. A. (1986) "A feminist perspective in midwifery", *Feminist Practice in Women's Healthcare*, Chichester: John Wiley & Sons, ed. Webb C.

p. 85 Office of Population Censuses and Surveys (1986) *Mortality Statistics, Perinatal and Infant: Social and Biological Factors*, Series DH3, London: HMSO, 17.

p. 86 WHO Regional Office for Europe (1986) adapted from *Having a Baby in Europe*, Copenhagen.
☐ Serkin M., Porte J. A., Monheit A. G. (May 1988) "The relationship of antepartum pelvic examinations to the incidence of premature rupture of the membranes, maternal

infection, and cesarean section", Paper given at the Scientific Session of Annual Clinical Meeting of American College of Obstetricians and Gynecologists.

p. 87 Pearce J. M., Campbell S. (1987) "A comparison of symphysis-fundal height and ultrasound as screening tests for light-for-gestational age infants", *British Journal of Obstetrics and Gynaecology*, 94, 100-104.
☐ Alexander S. *et al* (1989) "Biochemical assessment of fetal well-being", *Effective Care in Pregnancy and Childbirth*, 1, 455-476, eds. Chalmers I., Enkin M., Keirse M. J. N. C.
☐ Mohide P., Keirse M. J. N. C. (1989) "Biophysical assessment of fetal well-being", eds. Chalmers I., Enkin M., Keirse M. J. N. C., op. cit., 455-476.

p. 89 Robinson M. (1958) "Salt in pregnancy", *Lancet*, 1, 178-181.
☐ Rush D. (1989) "Effects of changes in protein and calorie intake during pregnancy on the growth of the human fetus", eds. Chalmers I., Enkin M., Keirse M. J. N. C., op. cit., 255-280.
☐ ibid.

p. 90 Priest J. (1990) *Drugs in Pregnancy*, London: Pandora, 99-101.
☐ McIntyre A. (1988) *Herbs for Pregnancy and Childbirth*, London: Sheldon.
☐ Hemminki E., Starfield B. (1985) "Routine administration of iron and vitamins during pregnancy: Review of controlled clinical trials", *British Journal of Obstetrics and Gynaecology*, 85, 404-410.
☐ Alexander S. *et al*, op. cit.

p. 110 Richards M., Dunn J., Antonis B. (1977) "Caretaking in the first year of life: The role of fathers' and mothers' social isolation", *Child Care Health Development*, 3, 23-36.

p. 112 Berry L. M. (1988) "Realistic expectation of the labor coach", *Journal of Obstetric Gynecologic and Neonatal Nursing*, 17, 5, 354-355.

p. 114 Perez P., Snedeker C. (1990) "Why parents need professional labor support", *Special Women*, Pennypress Inc.

p. 119 Kitzinger S. (1989) *Pregnancy and Childbirth*, London: Michael Joseph.

p. 124 Donnison J. (1990) *Midwives and Medical Men*, London: Heinemann.
☐ Pollock L. (1987) *A Lasting Relationship: Parents and Children over Three Centuries*, London: Fourth Estate.

p. 125 Mason J. (1988) quoting Miles L., "Pioneer Questionnaires (Health) SX-2" in "Midwifery in Canada", *The Midwife Challenge*, London: Pandora, ed. Kitzinger S.
☐ ibid.

p. 126 Benoit C. (Winter 1983) "Midwives and healers: The Newfoundland experience", *Health Sharing*, 22-25.
☐ ibid.
☐ Klaus M., Kennell J., Robertson S., Sosa R. (1986) "Effects of social support during parturition on maternal-infant morbidity", *British Medical Journal*, 293, 585-587.
☐ Hodnett E. D., Osborn R. W. (1989) "A randomized trial of the effects of monitrice support during labor: Mothers' views two to four weeks postpartum", *Birth*, 16, 4, 177-184.

p. 127 Flint C. (1986) *Sensitive Midwifery*, London: Heinemann.

p. 130 Kitzinger S., Nilsson L. (1986) *Being Born*, London: Dorling Kindersley.

p. 134 Rossavik I. K. (1989) *Obstetrics and Gynecology*, 73, 2, 243-249.
☐ Kramer M. S. (1988) *Journal of the American Medical Association*, 260, 22, 3306-3308.
☐ Lamont R. F. (1986) "Management of preterm labour", *Hospital Update*, 487-490, 492-493.
☐ Salmon Y. M. (1986) "Cervical ripening by breast stimulation", *Obstetrics and Gynecology*, 67, 1, 21-24; Curtis P. (1986) "Uterine responses to three techniques of breast stimulation", *Obstetrics and Gynecology*, 67, 1, 22-28; Curtis P. (1986) "Prepartum and intrapartum breast stimulation in obstetrics", *Journal of Reproductive Medicine*, 31, 4, 228-230.

p. 135 Eggersten S. C. (1987) "Maternal response to daily fetal movement counting in primary care settings", *American Journal of Perinatology*, 4, 4, 327-330.

p. 137 Steer P. J. (1986) "Postmaturity – much ado about nothing?", *British Journal of Obstetrics and Gynaecology*, 93, 2, 105-108; Yudkin P. L. (1986) "Caesarean section dissected 1978-1983", *British Journal of Obstetrics and Gynaecology*, 93, 2, 135-144; Cardozo L. (1986) "Prolonged pregnancy: The management debate", *British Medical Journal*, 293, 1059-1063.

p. 138 Sinquefield G. (1985) "Midwifery management of premature rupture of the membranes at term", *Journal of Nurse Midwifery*, 30, 4, 242-244.

☐ Lenihan J. P. (1984) "The relationship of antepartum pelvic examinations to premature rupture of the membranes", *Obstetrics and Gynecology*, 63, 33-37.

p. 139 Davis E. (1987) *Heart and Hands*, California: Celestial Arts.

p. 141 Butler N. R., Bonham D. G. (1963) *Perinatal Mortality*, Edinburgh: Churchill Livingstone.
☐ McKay S. (1983) "How worthwhile are membrane stripping and amniotomy?", *Contemporary Obstetrics and Gynecology*, 173-176, 178-181, 184.

p. 142 Newton N., Foshea D., Newton M. (1966) "Experimental inhibition of labor through environmental disturbance", *Obstetrics and Gynecology*, 67, 371-377.

p. 144 Salar G. *et al*, "Effect of transcutaneous electrotherapy on cerebro-spinal fluid beta-endorphin content in patients without pain problems", *Pain*, 10, 169-172; Polden M. (1985) "Transcutaneous nerve stimulation in labour and post-Caesarean section", *Physiotherapy*, 71, 8, 350-353.
☐ Harrison R. F. *et al* (1986) "Pain relief in labour using transcutaneous electrical nerve stimulation (TENS)", *British Journal of Obstetrics and Gynaecology*, 93, 7, 739, 746.

p. 146 Flint C., op. cit.
☐ Davis E., op. cit.
☐ Simkin P. (1989) *The Birth Partner*, The Harvard Common Press.

p. 148 Gaskin I. M. (1982) "Ask the midwives", *The Practicing Midwife*, 1, 15.

p. 150 Lawrence H. (1988) "Breathing for labour", *Journal of Association of Chartered Physiotherapists and Obstetrics in Gynaecology*, 60, 2, 21-23.
☐ Broach J., Newton N. (June 1988) "Food and beverages in labor. Part 1: Cross-cultural and historical practices. Part 2: The effects of cessation of oral intake during labor", *Birth*, 2, 15.
☐ Davis E., op. cit.

p. 152 Newton N., Foshea D., Newton M., op. cit.

p. 153 Cronk M., Flint C. (1989) *Community Midwifery: A Practical Guide*, London: Heinemann.
☐ Gaskin I. M. (1978) *Spiritual Midwifery*, Tennessee: The Book Publishing Co.

p. 154 Stein A. (1986) "Breech delivery: A co-operative nurse-midwifery medical management approach", *Journal of Nurse-Midwifery*, 31, 2, 93-97.
☐ Odent M. (1984) *Birth Reborn*, New York: Random House.

p. 155 Russell J. G. B. (1982) "The rationale of primitive delivery positions", *British Journal of Obstetrics and Gynaecology*, 89, 712-715.

p. 156 O'Leary J. A., Gunn D. L. (1986) "Option for shoulder dystocia: cephalic replacement", *Contemporary Obstetrics and Gynecology*, 27, 157.
☐ Gaskin I. M. (1988) "Shoulder dystocia: Controversies in management", *Birth Gazette*, 5, 1, 14-17.
☐ Flint C., op. cit.

p. 159 Davis E., op. cit.

p. 160 ibid.

p. 162 ibid.
☐ ibid.

p. 184 Leavitt J. W. (1986) *Brought to Bed: Childbearing in America 1750-1950*, New York: Oxford University Press.

p. 187 Winnicott D. J. (1964) *The Child, the Family, and the Outside World*, London: Penguin.

p. 189 Garforth S., Garcia J. (1989) "Breastfeeding policies and practice – 'no wonder they get confused'", *Midwifery*, 5, 2, 75-83.
☐ ibid.

p. 190 Kitzinger S. (1983) *The New Good Birth Guide*, London: Penguin, 139-142.
☐ Woolridge M. W. (1988) "Right from the start – establishing breastfeeding", Symposium on Caring for the Breastfeeding Mother, London: Kings Fund Centre.

p. 191 Office of Population Censuses and Surveys, Social Security Division (1988) *Infant feeding 1985*, London: HMSO.

p. 192 Kitzinger S. (1988) *Breastfeeding your Baby*, London: Dorling Kindersley.
☐ Pitt B. (1968) "Atypical depression following childbirth", *British Journal of Psychiatry*, 114, 1325-1335.

p. 193 Stein A. *et al* (1989) "Social adversity and perinatal complications: Their relation to postnatal depression", *British Medical Journal*, 290.
☐ Oakley A. (1980) *Women Confined*, Oxford: Martin Robertson.
☐ Affonso D. (1981) *Impact of Cesarean Childbirth*, Philadelphia: Davis; Bradley C. F. *et al* (1983) "A prospective study of mothers' attitudes and feelings following cesarean and vaginal births", *Birth* 10, 79-83; Garel M. *et al* (1987) "Psychological consequences of caesarean childbirth in primiparas", *Journal of Psychosomatic Obstetrics and Gynaecology*, 6, 197-209.
☐ Thune-Larsen K. B., Moller Pedersen K. (1988) "Childbirth experience and postpartum emotional disturbance", *Journal of Reproductive and Infant Psychology*, 6, 229-240.
☐ Entwistle D., Doering S. (1981) *The First Birth*, Baltimore: John Hopkins University Press; Green J., Coupland V., Kitzinger J. *Great Expectations* (based on research by Child Care Development Group, University of Cambridge), forthcoming; Kitzinger S. (1989) *The Crying Baby*, London: Penguin.
☐ Garel M. *et al*, op. cit.

INDEX

ACKNOWLEDGMENTS

Author's acknowledgments

I want to thank all those women who have described to me, often in great detail, their births and their feelings about them, those whose births I have been privileged to share, and the midwives who have explored their skills with me.

The women who were the subjects of the beautiful birth photographs in this book welcomed Marcia May into one of the most intimate experiences of their lives, because they wanted to show other women that birth outside the framework of a hospital was a positive experience. We both want to thank them very much.

My daughter, Tess, revealed to me through her labour the value of water births. I want to thank her for letting me participate in a birth that was different from, and longer and harder work than, my own births, but equally satisfying, when she gave birth to Sam, weighing 4.75kg (10½lb), triumphantly and without even tearing. The photographs of her birth were taken by my husband, who did this unobtrusively and with sensitivity.

The midwife friends who have advised me are Lesley Page, Director of Midwifery for Oxfordshire, who was one of Tess's two midwives, and Caroline Flint, initiator of the "Know your Midwife" scheme and Midwifery Consultant to the Riverside Health Authority in London. Although they are not responsible for what finally appears in print, I have learned a great deal from them.

I owe to my friend Penny Simkin, in Seattle, help with material about stress in childbirth and the action of catecholamines, as well as helpful discussions about the empowering of women in childbirth. I would also like to thank Dr Desmond Barden, consultant psychiatrist, and a warrior in the struggle for women's freedom in childbirth.

My daughter, Jenny, has added another dimension in discussing with me her research on midwives, doctors, and mothers' experiences, and both Jenny and another daughter, Polly, have widened my thinking about violence against women in childbirth because of their work with women who have been sexually abused.

There are very special women, many of them writers themselves, in different countries, with whom I value the opportunity to discuss birth issues, and who have helped me with my thinking on the theme of this book. They include Jan Brandt in Uppsala, Dr Ann Oakley and Wendy

Savage FRCOG in London, Laura Cao Romero de Abascal in Mexico City, Dr Jo Garcia and Jean Robinson in Oxford, Doris Haire in New York and Norma Swenson in Boston, Dr Ulla Waldenstrom in Stockholm, Dr Mary O'Brien in Toronto, as well as courageous groups of home birth midwives in the United States, Canada, Scandinavian countries, Germany, Austria, Switzerland, Spain, Italy, Australia, New Zealand, and Britain. My warmest thanks to them all.

Although it took me a long time to think through, this book was completed in record time because of the hard work of Kim Hamilton and Rosie Campbell, who applied themselves to the wordprocessor with unfailing good humour and lively interest in the subject matter. I am enormously grateful to each of them.

Publisher's acknowledgments

Dorling Kindersley would like to thank Rosalind Priestley for seeing the book through all stages of production; Laura Harper for her editorial help; Vanessa Hamilton for her design help, and Hilary Bird for the index.

All photographs are by Marcia May except those on pages 178-181, which are by Uwe Kitzinger, and the portrait of the author on the jacket flap, which is by Nancy Durrell McKenna.